# A Wa

A Story of cour
a stage 4 Breast Cancer Survivor!

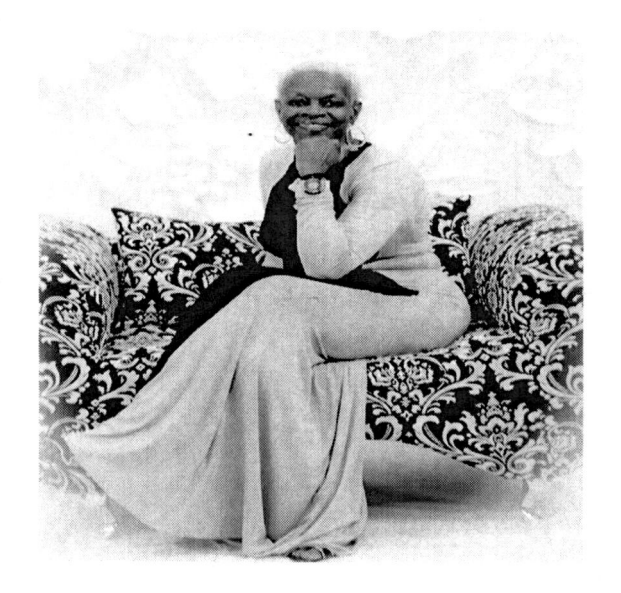

*Patricia Johnson*

Copyright © 2014
by
Patricia Johnson

All rights reserved. No part of this publication may be reproduced, distributed, or transmitted in any form or by any means, including photocopying, recording, or other electronic or mechanical methods, without the prior written permission of the author or publisher, except in the case of brief quotations embodied in critical reviews and certain other noncommercial uses permitted by copyright law.

ISBN #978-0-983583066

Library of Congress Cataloging
in-Publication Data

Johnson, Patricia

First Printing 2014
Edited by Dr. Mia Y. Merritt

Printed in the U.S.A.

## Introduction

Writing this book was like dissecting myself piece by piece. As I wrote this book, I had to relive my deepest feelings, fears, discouragements, doubts and frustrations as I reached deep within to pull those emotions out. The most liberating part of it all is that the other side of those negative emotions was courage, faith, joy, peace and the motivation that I could and would beat cancer. My desire is for others to read my book and dissect themselves, so they can realize that they have the power within to beat and overcome any challenge that comes their way. This power is given to them of God. It's a good thing for the soul to be refreshed as your spirit is elevated and uplifted. Experiences in life come and go, and with each new experience, a wise lesson is left behind. My heart is filled with gratitude for the smallest things now that I have overcome this enormous fight with breast cancer. If writing this book will help only one person, then my writing was not in vain because I have done what I was asked to do by my Master.

When the Holy Spirit said to me, *"Write a book"* I tried to push it away, thinking, *I don't know how to write a book.* I had no idea where to start. That very same night, I was awakened at 2:00a.m. by the Holy Spirit speaking to me to take each letter in the word "family" and make a word. I laid there thinking where is this message coming from? My mind quickly started to work, F A M I L Y! What can I do with this? As I pondered, I realized that the letters in this word are what helped me to get healed. Had it not been for these things, I would not have been able to make it through as courageously and miraculously as I did:

| | |
|---|---|
| **F** | Friends & faith |
| **A** | Attitude |
| **M** | Miracles |
| **I** | Inspiration |
| **L** | Love |
| **Y** | Yield |

As I look at the words beside each letter, I see that I needed them all. Thank you Holy Spirit for helping me to see that my "family" consisted of friends, faith, attitude, miracles, inspiration, love and my yielding to you.

My dear family and friends, there will be people who do not understand your God given role. And that is okay. You are not called to please them. You are called to please God, So do not be ashamed if your God-given assignment is outside of the realms of the norm. Just do what God has called you to do. If God has spoken to you, it's up to you to answer what He has asked you to do. Be joyous everyday working toward the plan He has for you. His plan for your life is marvelous. It is grand and it is great!

# Dedication

I dedicate this book to everyone who spoke positive, uplifting words into my spirit during the hardest time of my life. Being told that I had stage four breast cancer and then told that the cancer was in my left breast, my spine, my hip, and my lymph nodes was devastatingly painful to hear. However, I was constantly strengthened and lifted up by the prayers of those who love and care for me. Family and friends are a gift from God, and I thank Him for the many gifts I have.

I would like to publicly thank my loving husband Charles, who never left my side and who continues to uplift and support me daily. He calls and checks on me every day. His love and encouragement, made my healing easier to manifest. I love him with all my heart.

God has blessed me with a beautiful church family who epitomizes and exemplifies the love of Christ. My brothers and sisters of Trinity Church in Miami Gardens, Florida embraced me, loved me, prayed for me, and labored with me during my fight against breast cancer. My pastor, Rich Wilkerson Sr. and his beautiful wife Robyn adopted me in the spirit and never ceased praying for me. They made me realize that I was loved, and that they were there for me until the end. My heart thanks God almighty for faithful servants such as the two of them who know how to gently care for and love the sheep of God.

To my sons, my sisters, and my girlfriends, I thank God for each of you. I love you, and I am so glad to have you all in my life. There is a special place inside my heart for each of you.

# Table of Contents

Chapter 1: The day my Life Shifted ...............................................1

Chapter 2: Faith, the Evidence ....................................................23

Chapter 3: Your Attitude has Power ............................................49

Chapter 4: Faithful Family ...........................................................77

Chapter 5: Comforting words for the Soul................................101

Chapter 6: Men and Breast Cancer ...........................................123

Prayer for Cancer .......................................................................132

Scriptures for Healing ................................................................135

About the Author .......................................................................138

# Chapter 1
## The Day My Life Shifted

As I was writing this book, I pondered upon the things that I survived through that others did not. I'm grateful because I am a cancer survivor! The beginning of the journey that would birth my awesome testimony started on July 3, 2008 when my Gynecologist's office called me to inform me that my mammogram showed something abnormal in my left breast. An appointment for a biopsy was made immediately and another one was made to see the breast surgeon. As I was listening to the medical assistant give me the results of my mammogram over the phone, my heart stopped beating, and I felt that my life, as I knew it, was over. I had always been good about having my mammograms each year from the time that I turned 40, and then consistently each year thereafter, so understandably I was confused because I thought I had done all the right things. This could not be happening to me. Why me? Many questions raced through my mind. Where did I go wrong? Why this news this time of

*The day my Life Shifted*

my life? What was the abnormality in the breast? What's going to happen to me? I was afraid, but also puzzled because I had experienced no pain in my breasts at all. I had never felt any lumps, had no rashes, there was no dripping, and my nipples were fine. I had been good about performing my own exams while in the shower, so the logical conclusion in my mind was that the doctor's office had somehow made an error. Yes, that was it. They had made a mistake. However, I went in to have the biopsy done as I was told. When my husband and I walked into the room where the technician was, I could see my x-rays up on the projector. The technician looked at me and said, *"Pat, I think its cancer."* This was told to me even before I had the biopsy. The x-rays were clear and it appeared to be obvious to the technician that what she saw was cancer. I kept calm and began asking questions. I went from one question to the next. Since I had a girlfriend who had gone through the breast cancer process, I knew exactly what questions to ask.

I had been in frequent conversations with my friend Sabrina after her biopsy, her diagnosis, the chemotherapy, her surgery, and eventually when she had to undergo a mastectomy; so I was pretty on top of just what to ask. After the technician had answered all of my questions, she asked my husband to leave the room so that she could prepare me for the biopsy. After he left the room, I broke down. I was afraid because when you hear that you have cancer, you immediately look at the diagnosis as your death sentence. The time after the biopsy and the official diagnosis was scary. I had to wait a whole week until I would know something for sure. I was trying to resolve in my mind that I was okay and that maybe what they saw was just cysts in my breasts. I tried to make myself feel better, but deep down inside, I could feel that something was not right, and I was worried.

### You Have Cancer

It seemed like forever, but I saw the breast surgeon a week later. At this time, I did not know the results of my biopsy, but unbeknownst to me, the surgeon had received the results already. He informed me that the results had confirmed that I did have stage two breast cancer, but that he would be able to perform a lumpectomy surgery, where they would simply go in and remove the cancer and the area where it started. I had some knowledge of what a lumpectomy was since Sabrina had gone through it. As she was experiencing her challenge with breast cancer, I did my research on it, so that I could understand all that she was undergoing. Little did I know, I would need that same research for myself. The tumor was under my left arm in my lymph nodes, and it was about two centimeters long. The surgeon explained to me that a lumpectomy surgery was a common surgical procedure designed to remove a lump for a malignant tumor. He proceeded to say that the tissue removed would be somewhat limited and that the procedure was relatively non-invasive compared to a mastectomy. With a lumpectomy, my breast would be preserved. With a mastectomy, they would have been removed. There was no lump in my left breast, but there were calcifications in it which spread to the breasts from the lump under the arm. Calcifications are tiny flecks of calcium such as grains of salt in the soft tissue of the breast that most times indicate the presence of breast cancer. Calcifications cannot be felt, but they do appear on mammograms. The surgeon further explained that I needed to make an appointment with my primary care physician, so that I could get pre-oped for surgery. I did that, but before having surgery, I was sent to get bone scans, cat scans, MRI's, and pelvic biopsies. The purpose of having those additional tests and x-rays was to ensure that the cancer was not also in other places of my body. While there with him, he noticed that my neck looked a little swollen and questioned me about it. I told him that I had always had that, so he dismissed it and that was that.

    After I had gone to all of the specialists that I was told to see, I went back to my surgeon to review all of the results and to discuss the specifics of the impending lumpectomy surgery. For some reason, when I arrived, I could sense that something was wrong. The doctor's disposition towards me seemed to be different. When it was time to talk to me, I was in the examining room and the nurse was standing closely beside me. I noticed that the surgeon would not come completely in the room, but he was standing at the entrance of the door and began talking to me from there. He began by saying, *Pat, you are not a stage two, you are a stage four. Cancer was found in some other areas of your body. We found cancer in your left breast, your spine, the left hip, and in your lymph nodes under your left arm.* He then explained that he would not be able to do the lumpectomy anymore, but that I would have to eventually have a mastectomy after going through chemotherapy and radiation. Needless-to-say, I completely broke down in that doctor's office. I could not believe what my ears had just heard. Everything seemed to be surreal. I thought I was having a bad dream, more like a nightmare. At that point, I

*The day my Life Shifted*

lost physical strength and could barely sit up. A hundred different thoughts raced through my mind, but at the same time, I could not think straight. Among other things, I thought, "Am I going to die so young? I am not strong enough to live with cancer, nor do I have the courage to wait for a cure. Why Lord? Why me? Why me? Why me! I wept and wailed. This was the worst day of my life! While going through my brake down, I heard the doctor ask the nurse, *Did she faint?* She said, *No she didn't.* She was still standing beside me, holding me. That was the reason she had been standing so close to me from the beginning. I assume that they were used to the reactions of women after being given their diagnosis, so she was there to catch me if I fell. The nurse then told the doctor, *We need to get the psychologist in here.* Before she left the room, she asked my husband Charles to come take her place and hold me in case I fainted; so he came and held me. Charles and I were left in the room and there was complete silence. He was quiet and so was I. Shortly thereafter, a young, pretty, well-dressed Anglo woman entered the room. She

> *Among other things, I thought, "Am I going to die so young? I'm not strong enough to live with cancer nor do I have the courage to wait for a cure. Why Lord? Why me? Why me? Why me!"*

approached me, stood in front of me and just looked into my eyes for about 20-30 seconds. She did not say a word to me. She just looked at me. Finally, she said, *What are you thinking?* and I said, *I'm going to die.* She said, *No, you are not going to die.* Yes I am. I said. *Cancer has spread all throughout my body and I'm gonna die!* Then she stated, *Listen to me. You are NOT going to die. If they felt that there was nothing they could do for you, they would have told you that. They are obligated by law to tell you if that were the case.* Then I said, *My sisters are not here. Both my mother and father are dead. I have nobody!* She then looked at my husband and pointed, then said, *Who is that?* I looked over at him. He was slumped down in the chair as though the life had been taken out of his body. He had pulled out his handkerchief and was quietly sobbing. So I looked back at her and said, *Look at him. How can he help me? Look at him! He's broken down like me.* So she said, *But he's here.* And for some reason, that actuality gave me a calmness and made me feel that yes, somebody was there for me - my husband of then 29 years. After she had finished counseling me, uplifting me, and giving me hope, I sat there and tried to wrap my head around all that was happening. My husband eventually said, *Tricia, we need to go.* I had just been sitting there in that room with no strength or motivation to even move. I finally got up and we walked out. To lighten the mood, my husband looked at me and said, *Tricia, now don't you embarrass me by fainting in this place.* I then burst into laughter and he started laughing as well. The receptionist at the front desk and those nearby asked what was so funny. I told them what my husband had just said to me and they said, *Now we need to hit him.* My husband had managed to turn my emotions of deep sorrow and fear into a lighthearted laughter. I needed that at that moment and I appreciate him for that. It mattered so much that day.

## Renewed Hope

After I regained my composure, I discovered an inner peace that I cannot explain with words. I remembered my granddaughter Charlese (a.k.a. Cha Chi) who is my heart's delight. I had promised to get her violin lessons and I had to keep that promise. In those few moments of clarity, I resolved to never give up. Hope was born in me. I decided to fight for my life with every fiber of my being and I never thought twice about the decision I had just made to fight. I became determined to live each moment to the fullest as I grabbed hold of my inner self to carry me through what was clearly turning into a traumatic experience.

When I made it home that day, the first person I told about my diagnosis was my youngest sister Yvonne, since she lives closest to me. My other two sisters live out of town, so I told them later that week. I did not tell many people initially, but after informing my sisters, I then informed my closest friends. I was blessed with a network of supporting friends, sisters, and family members who encouraged me daily. Through their love, support, and constant uplifting, I was able to face my fears with a blessed hope for my future. My friend Sabrina of whom I have referenced had already gone through what I was now facing. She was insistent in coming to me from Atlanta, GA to accompany me to my first oncologist appointment. I told her that she did not have to come because my husband would be there with me. Her reply to me was, *Charles doesn't have breasts!* I am going with you! She then told me what date she would be flying in and what time she would need to be picked up from the airport. No questions asked. Well, I guess that settled that!

### The White Horse

After receiving the devastating news that I had gone from a stage two to a stage four, I had to go home and collect myself. I had to find a place of being able to process all that was happening to me. I needed God. I needed Him badly and

*The day my Life Shifted*

I needed Him NOW. I engrossed myself with busyness. I prayed. I cried. I tried to remain strong for my husband and my children, but on the inside I was scared. The time came for me to see the oncologist for the first time. I went to bed that night prepared for the appointment, but I could not sleep. It was about 2:00a.m in the morning, so I decided to get up and get into my jacuzzi to relax and pray. When I got in and relaxed my body, I looked up at the sky. With wide-opened eyes looking upward, I suddenly had an open vision. As clear as day, I saw a beautiful white stallion, and riding on the stallion was me! I had on a white sheer-flowing dress, and riding with me were four other women. Two were riding on the left of me and two were on the right of me. Their horses were darker colored. I was in the middle and was the only one with a white horse. All of us were galloping fast, seemingly chasing away someone on another horse. I could see a man in front of us running away with a frightening look on his face. That was all I saw. Just as quick as I saw the vision, it disappeared. After seeing that, I was in a state of disbelief. I had never in my life had a vision, or had I ever seen anything like that. Once I gathered my thoughts, I received the vision as confirmation that I was going to be healed. I interpreted the vision to mean that I and the angels of God were chasing away the devil. A sense of peace came over me and I knew in my soul that I was going to be just fine. God had just shown me that I was in His hands and He loved me enough to send angels to help me fight my battle. A few days later, I looked up the meaning of a white horse and this is what I found:

*The rider of a white horse goes out "conquering and to conquer" and **does not lose a battle**. He is victorious in all encounters with the enemy. As he goes out to conquer, he has definite objectives to accomplish his conquering.*

From that moment on, I no longer went to my appointments discouraged or afraid because I knew what I knew. I had enough wisdom to know that I needed to do my part on this side of heaven, but I also knew in my heart what the end result was going to be. I went to bed, got up a few hours later, and headed for my appointment with the oncologist.

## Starting Treatments

On the day of my appointment with the oncologist, my sister had arranged for an entourage consisting of her and my close friends to accompany me to the doctor. I had just had my vision the night before, and although I knew that the women on the horses represented God's war angels, I also

*The day my Life Shifted*

looked at my entourage of family and friends as those women on the horses. They were also my angels on earth. This was an interesting day because seven people including my husband escorted me to my first oncologist appointment. Each had a pad and pen that my sister had given them to ask questions and take notes.

While speaking with the oncologist, the first question I asked was when I was going to start my chemotherapy and radiation treatments. Her response to me was shocking. She said, *We will not be doing any of that. Nor will you be having a mastectomy.* Confused, I said, *But the surgeon told me that I would have to have a mastectomy, undergo chemotherapy and have radiation.* And she said, *I am your cancer doctor and the surgeon is a man. Surgeons always want to cut. I am not going to take your body through those extreme measures if I don't have to. We are going to try something else first and that is a pill called Femara . Since your body is estrogen sensitive, this pill blocks estrogen from spreading.* I had found out that my body produces a lot of estrogen, which is what caused the cancer to spread in various parts. The Femara blocks the body from producing estrogen. Estrogen and cancer do not mix. It's like oil and water. A week later, I returned to my oncologist for my first treatment, and to pick

*A Walking Miracle!*

up my prescription for the Femara. As my husband was driving up, I saw in big bold letters on top of the building, the words CANCER CENTER. It then became real for me. I said to myself, *When I walk in there, everyone's going to know that I have cancer.* It was not a good feeling for me that day. I saw so many people who looked so sick. You could see it all over them. I thought to myself that at some point, I was going to start looking like that too. I was scared, discouraged, and deeply disheartened that day.

    They finally called me to have my blood drawn. As I sat there, I began sobbing. The reality of it all began to sink in. When I finished having the blood drawn, I went into the next area to wait for the doctor to come in. Eventually my oncologist entered, reviewed my blood work with me, talked to me about the intravenous treatment that I was going to start getting, then told me that she wanted me to schedule an appointment to have a biopsy done on my left hip. Although the surgeon had confirmed that the cancer had spread to my left hip, she wanted to be double sure before she began the treatment in that area. After we were done, I headed for my first treatment. As I walked in the treatment room, I saw many patients receiving their chemotherapy. Everyone was hooked up to IVs, some who were too sick to sit up were

*The day my Life Shifted*

lying down, but I could see it all. I could not believe that I was there to receive a treatment for cancer. Although I was not getting a chemotherapy treatment, I received an intravenous medication called Zometa. This medication helped to keep my bones strong since the cancer was also in my bones. I only needed to return every six weeks for blood work, to receive the Zometa treatment, and to see the doctor. The Femara , which was my other medication was a pill that I took once a day to block my body from producing estrogen. The process of going in every six weeks was always the same. They drew blood, the oncologist came in to speak with me, then I went and received treatments. I thought that at some point, I would begin feeling weak and tired from the treatments, but to my surprise, I was just fine. I was energetic, continued doing my normal routines, and was never sick one day as a result of my treatments. In fact, if I would not have gotten my mammogram that year, I would not have known that anything was wrong with me. As mentioned before, I had no pain, no rashes, and there was never any lump that I was able to feel when I would do my own breast exams. I have always exercised by walking and lifting weights and maybe that was why the treatments did not affect my energy level.

*A Walking Miracle!*

After returning the second time, the oncologist reviewed the results of my hip biopsy. Strangely, it came back negative, and she was not satisfied at those results. She said to me, *Pat, although the hip biopsy came back negative, I am 95% sure that it is cancer. I think that because the cancer is so small, he may have missed it. Would you mind having another hip biopsy done?* I said to her, *Dr. Krill, I will do anything you ask me to do, but I want you to know that I am healed. God has healed me.* As requested, I had the second biopsy done, and again, the results came back negative, so when I saw my oncologist for my third treatment, I said, *See, I told you that I have been healed.* Those negative results gave me a sense of hope that I would be fine. Because of my vision, I felt and believed that eventually no cancer would be found in any area of my body. Despite how I felt on my first day going to the cancer center, God replaced my feelings of deep sadness and fear with peace and joy. He reminded me of the vision I had in the jacuzzi and put a strong conviction in me that I was going to be just fine. It was the enemy trying to get me to focus on my situation in the natural, but in reality, God had me in His hands and in His timing, my healing would come.

*The day my Life Shifted*

**The Male Peacock**

At first I didn't understand why this was happening to me, but when God gave me peace and joy in the midst of my challenges, I knew that it was for a bigger cause that He had predestined for me from the foundation of the world. Knowing that this was part of His plan for my life, gave me peace and assurance. I knew that my experience would birth a great testimony, and now it has birthed this book. To God be the glory! In the meantime, my body was responding well to both the Femara (for blocking the estrogen) and the Zometa (to strengthen my bones). The time between each treatment had me constantly taking tests. About three months after receiving treatments, I had a PET scan done. This is a machine that uses radiation or nuclear medicine imaging to produce 3-dimensional color images of the functional processes within the human body. PET stands for *positron emission tomography*. It was used to diagnose or rediagnose my condition, to find out how my body was developing and to see how effective the treatments were. The PET scan revealed that tumors were shrinking and even disappearing! The cancer found in my spine and pelvic bone had disappeared. The lymph nodes had shrunk from a size eight to a size two, and the cancer in my left breast was diminishing.

*A Walking Miracle!*

I continued with my treatments every six weeks, and also my daily dose of Femara , which I still take to this very day. Although the cancer in my body was almost gone, my oncologist informed me that I must still have surgery to remove the tiny bit of cancer that was still left in my left breast. This was where the cancer had originally started. This surgery would be a lumpectomy surgery. Initially, I started off being told that I would only need a lumpectomy, only to be told later on that I had to have a mastectomy. Now I was being told again that all I needed was a lumpectomy. God was moving in my life in a mighty and mysterious way, and I was grateful. I could see His hand in all of this. I was happy and full of joy. I felt like a male peacock because the male is much prettier than the female. He's a beautiful creation of God, definitely a sight to behold. His tail feathers are colored green, blue, and orange. Besides the blue peacocks, there are also green peacocks with golden-green bodies and necks. Both kinds have been bred to have many different colors of feathers including white. In spite of what I was going through, I felt beautiful, vibrant, and confident because I knew that my Father was with me and that He was working all things out for my good.

*The day my Life Shifted*

## The Lumpectomy Surgery

I returned to the surgeon to discuss the lumpectomy surgery, which I had the very next month. After the surgery, I was told that 17 of my lymph nodes had been removed. Lymph nodes are part of the lymphatic system, which connected to the immune system that helps filter bacteria and cancer cells from the body. The lymph nodes, which are located in many areas of the body including the neck, the armpit, the groin, under the jaw, the back of the head and other places, produce immune cells that help the body fight infection. Because they help to filter cancer out of the body, they may become cancerous if there is a mass nearby that is attempting to spread through the body. Lymph nodes may be swollen when fighting bacteria or disease. When they become swollen and tender, their location is far more obvious, leading some people to say that their glands are swollen. The human body consists of 20 to 30 lymph nodes in your arm. Two of my lymph nodes were cancerous.

After the lumpectomy surgery, I came home the same day. Nurses came in to help show me how to drain the fluid from under my arm. Physical Therapists came in to help me strengthen my arm. Two and ½ months later, I was back to work! I had a team of good doctors who genuinely cared for me and were concerned about my health and my well-being.

*A Walking Miracle!*

While I was recuperating at home, I began writing my testimony. I then made copies and began giving them to everyone I saw. Upon returning to Delta Airlines as a flight attendant, I approached my supervisor and said to her, *I want to be in the Sky Delta Magazine next month in October for Breast Cancer Month.* Her response to me was, *"Ok Pat. Let me find out who I need to call and I'll get back with you.* About two weeks later, I received a call from the Assistant Editor of the magazine. She told me that she had my testimony on her desk and that I would be in October's edition of Sky Magazine. I was elated because I knew that my testimony was going all over the world, since Delta Airlines flies everywhere. What the devil meant for evil, God worked out for my good!

While I was in Sky Magazine, I was still receiving treatments, but my body was responding excessively well to the medication. I was about 85% cancer free and was well on my way to being 100% cancer free! I had such a positive attitude and knew that God was using me to spread the Word of His goodness, but the enemy of my faith would not let me be completely healed without a fight. My swollen thyroids continued to bother the surgeon. He wanted to ensure that everything in my throat area was okay because the size of

*The day my Life Shifted*

my glands looked abnormal to him, so he requested a biopsy. The biopsy results revealed that my cells were abnormal, so he immediately requested surgery to remove my thyroids. They only had to remove one thyroid because the other one was fine. After the surgery, I could not talk for three months. I whispered everything I had to say. I could not go to work during this time because I needed my voice to speak to passengers and shout commands in the event of an emergency. I was extremely frustrated during this time. When the speech therapist told me that I may never get my voice back, my heart dropped to my stomach, but shortly thereafter, I remembered whose hands my health was in, and from that moment on, my faith led me to believe that I would get my voice back, and I did. It took three months, but my sexy voice did come back and I did not have to take any thyroid medication resulting from the surgery. My one remaining thyroid is functioning at maximum capacity and my throat area is just fine.

After overcoming the thyroid surgery, I was back to work, and continued to spread the goodness of God and how

*A Walking Miracle!*

He had healed me from cancer. By this time, I was about 90% cancer free and six-months later, there was no more cancer to be found in my body! I am 100% cancer free! Although I am a cancer survivor, I still take the Femara daily because it stops my body from producing estrogen, which feeds cancer; and I continue to receive Zometa treatments once a year to keep my bones strengthened. From the day that I was diagnosed to this very day, I had a journey that consisted of shock, disappointment, fear, discouragement, frustration, faith, joy, peace, love for God and now extreme gratitude and praise for what He has done for me. In order to come out of anything victoriously, you must believe by faith that God will help you get through it. You must embrace an attitude of gratitude!

### POINTS TO PONDER

> God had just shown me that I was in His hands and He loved me enough to send angels to help me fight my battle.

- I felt like a male peacock, because the male is much prettier than the female. He's a beautiful creation of God, definitely a sight to behold!

- I was so happy because I knew that my testimony was going all over the world, since Delta Airlines flies everywhere!

- I became determined to live each moment to the fullest as I grabbed hold of my inner self to carry me through what was clearly turning into a traumatic experience.

# Chapter 2
# Faith

*But without faith it is impossible to please* him: *for he that cometh to* God *must believe that he is, and that he is a rewarder of them that diligently seek Him.* ~Hebrews 11:6

Without faith, it is impossible to please God (Hebrews 11:6). In order to believe that God will heal you of whatever affliction you have, you must have faith. Faith is knowing beyond a shadow of a doubt that the outcome is going to be just fine - even if the situation in the natural realm looks hopeless and grim. Faith is believing that substance is there when there is no sign of substance in the physical realm. *Now faith is the substance of things hoped for, the evidence of things not seen (Hebrews 11:1).* Your faith is your evidence. Faith is believing that whatever you are trusting God for already exists in the spiritual realm and you are simply waiting for the manifestation in the natural realm. In order to remain strong and totally trust God, I had to learn to exercise my faith every day. I had to walk it out and believe

*Faith*

that God was watching and protecting me. Being a flight attendant for many years forced me to have faith in the pilots with my life as they would fly the airplanes. I had to believe that they would get us to each destination safely. I had to have faith in their abilities. Without doubting and questioning, I believed that everything would be okay while we were up in the air because it always had been. It is the same with God. Without doubting and questioning, I had to trust that everything would be just fine with my health, because it always had been. Why do we sometimes have more faith in people and things than we do in God? Things in my life had always turned out fine for me, so I had to have faith that this was no different.

Elisabeth Elliot said, *"True faith only goes into operation when there are no answers."* God says, my thoughts are not your thoughts, nor are your ways my ways (Isaiah. 55:8). God doesn't think like us. He sees the big picture and works toward specific ends. He looks at everything from the realm of eternity. Just know He's always watching. Nothing escapes Him. He knows everything that is going on with you and He has a divine plan for your glorious future. Just continue praising Him, glorifying Him, honoring Him, and sharing His Word. If you are faithful to Him, He will be faithful to you! When you doubt your faith, pray. Hannah Whitall Smith said that faith is the simplest, plainest thing in the world. It's simply believing God for what you feel, think, or wish for. It is simply a matter of believing in Him; so I choose to doubt my doubts and believe in Him.

### Trusting God

Being diagnosed with stage four breast cancer put me in an unfamiliar place because I needed to put my whole faith in God, the invisible One. I couldn't see Him physically the way I could see and touch the airplane pilots who I had faith in, but I had to trust Him the same way I trusted them. I was however, able to feel God with me. I cannot see the wind either, but I can feel it blow pass me, therefore, I know it's there. The evidence that the wind is there is when I see leaves moving on the trees. When I feel love, courage, and faith spring up in me, that's evidence that

*Faith*

God is there. Faith has filled and built my heart with trust and strength. Since I allowed faith to be a guiding motivating factor in my life, I have a new outlook. When I cried out to God to heal me, I believed He would. I had no doubt. He always comes through for His faithful children. He never leaves us nor forsakes us (Hebrews 13:5).

As hard as life can be sometimes, the reality of it all is that we must face our challenges head on. We must learn to hold our heads up high and have the grace, dignity, and assurance that everything will be all right; so the next time your life starts to feel like a roller coaster ride, climb into the front seat, not the back, not the middle, but the front seat; throw your hands high in the air, then enjoy the ride! We must understand that problems force us to look to God and depend on Him instead of trying to depend upon ourselves.

I did not know having cancer would bring so many chapters in my life, but it did. I thank God for the new chapters because I have learned to find the good in every situation. If I can find the good in having stage four breast cancer, then you certainly can find the good in your situation. Each situation brings us closer to God. He is your strength, your peace, your joy, your doctor, your everything.

## Women and Faith

On January 15, 2010, my cousin died from breast cancer. At the time, I was still getting my treatments. When I first heard the news, I sobbed. As I reflect back, I am not sure if I was sobbing from the loss of my cousin's life or because I felt that I was next. Fear overtook me because I was still fighting the disease and going to treatments. Looking back now, I know that it is human nature to become fearful when you hear of someone passing away from the same thing that you have. The first thing that comes to mind is, "Am I next?" Although I grieved for my cousin and attended her funeral, I did not let fear grip me as it was trying to. I prayed about it and released it. I remember apologizing to God for feeling that way, and I said to Him, "God, cancer scares me." However, I continued holding on to my faith and belief that I would be healed.

*Faith*

### Tonya, my Guardian Angel

Meeting Tonya Ferguson was not by chance. People come into our lives for a reason, a season or a lifetime. When we figure out their purpose for entering out lives, we will know exactly what to do. There is no such thing as coincidences. Every encounter we have is by divine appointment. That is how I met Tonya, by divine appointment. After I had been healed from stage four breast cancer, I promised God that I would share His goodness with every person I met, and I did. I typed my story and testimony of how God had healed me. I had it laminated and made plenty of copies. As my spirit led me, I gave copies to anyone who would listen. One day while in Dunkin Doughnuts, I began talking to the young girls who worked there about the importance of getting their mammograms; and I gave them a copy of my testimony. One of the workers said to me, *"I have a stepsister who has cancer. Is it okay if I give her your contact information?* Of course I agreed. When Tonya (the stepsister), called me, we immediately bonded. We talked and prayed together for hours that first day. Tonya was a beautiful 30-year-old young lady who had been

*A Walking Miracle!*

diagnosed with stage four breast cancer. She had two children, ages 11 and 16 at the time. The cancer had spread to both of her breasts, her sternum, lungs, and bones. From the time we met, we talked every single day. Then one day I asked her if she would like me to accompany her to chemotherapy, and she said yes. The next week, I drove her to her treatments and met her mother the same day. That day, my world changed completely. To see someone so young and in so much physical and mental anguish was extremely disheartening for me. It was my first day seeing Tonya face-to-face, but she wanted me right there by her side because of the bond we had shared in the spirit. While at the doctors, Tonya asked me to go in as she talked to her oncologist. When she took off her shirt for the oncologist to examine her breasts, I saw how the cancer had horribly disfigured her chest. My heart bled for Tonya. I was grateful that she trusted me enough to allow me into the room, but I was also grateful to know that Tonya knew I would love her in spite of it all. God had appointed me to be with her, and I made a vow that I would be there for her no matter what. She and I

*Faith*

spent a lot of time talking on the phone and texting. She began introducing me to her family and friends as her "guardian angel", but I would respond back and tell her that *she* was *my* angel. While with me, Tonya managed to laugh and talk to me about a variety of things. Through all of her pain and cancer prognosis, she knew that God loved her. On my days off, I would go and visit her. Her mother was extremely appreciative because she had to work and was grateful that I could be there with Tonya on the days that she was working. Her mother was always there by her daughter's side when she was off. Tonya had a close-knit family. She was never alone. There was never a time that I went to see her that one of her family members was not there by her side; and I fell right on in as though I were one of the family members. They embraced and loved me as such. Sometimes I would go to Tonya's house and just sit with her; other times I would go over and make her some soup; still other times I would put a hot towel on her back. Since the cancer had gotten into her bones and had spread over her body, it caused pain in her back, so the hot towel gave her a little

*A Walking Miracle!*

comfort. Every day, we would sing 'Jesus loves me, this I know'. If she had a treatment on my day off, I would take her to it and if not, I would just spend time with her at her house. I once took her to the beach for a nice outing. Because of her oxygen tank and her getting tired, we could not walk all the way to the shore, so we sat in the sand. I walked to the ocean with a bucket, filled it up, brought it back to where Tonya was, and poured it on her legs. I had always heard that salt water was healing, and that's why I did it. She laughed and said

> *"Tonya was like a daughter to me, although she had a devoted and sweet mother of her own. Every night we would text each other to say goodnight and to say I love you. Our time together was precious."*

that it was cold, but she loved it. That was a special moment for us. We even took pictures that day. We were a blessing to each other. With Tonya, I forgot about myself, or what may have been going on with me at the time, because she was my priority when I was with her. I had spiritually adopted her as my daughter and had placed her in a special place inside my heart. I would often hold her hand and let her know that she had to live for today and put tomorrow into God's hands. I

*Faith*

taught her to cherish each moment and live for that moment. We do not have any control when it comes to birth or death, but we do have control with what we do in between.

Although Tonya had a devoted and sweet mother, I looked to her as my very child. Every night we would text each other to say goodnight and I love you. Our time together was precious. Tonya became the daughter I never had and her family became my family. As the days and months passed, Tonya's cancer was not reacting to the chemotherapy or radiation anymore. It became extremely aggressive and metastasized in her body. The doctors finally told her that there was nothing else they could do. Her mother and I took her records to another medical facility for a second opinion, and were told the same thing. While I was at Tonya's home one day, she said to me, *"Come here Ms. Pat"* so I approached her as she was sitting up at the head of the bed. Then she told me to come closer. Before she began speaking to me, she was so close that we could almost touch each other's noses. Then, she said to me in a very courageous way, *"I'm not scared. I just don't want to leave my daughters."* All I could think of to say at the moment

*A Walking Miracle!*

was, *"I know Tonya. They are going to be alright."* Before going to spend time with her on my days off, I would pray and ask God for strength to be a help to her and to give me the right words to say. I would daily listen to a song by Yolanda Adams entitled 'I'm Gonna be Ready' to prepare my heart and mind to be with Tonya. I knew that I did not have any power over her situation, but I had power over what role I would play in her life. I had power over how I would make her feel. I had power over taking care of one of God's children that He assigned to me, and I was going to do that to the best of my ability. It is our duty to fulfill whatever assignment that God gives to each of us. I had to stay strong and cherish each moment I had with Tonya. When it got to the point where time was winding down, I was asked by Tonya's mother not to come to the hospital anymore because they were only keeping her sedated. She was in a deep sleep around the clock. At that point, whoever entered Tonya's hospital room had to wear a facemask and gloves. Because of the fact that I had previously been diagnosed with breast cancer, it was best for me not to go back into the room.

*Faith*

Tonya had degenerated so badly that it was not good for others to see her that way. Her mother was also concerned that I would become too distraught to see Tonya in the condition that she had slipped into so quickly. She was concerned that the stress would not be good for a breast cancer survivor. Of course, I honored the request and stayed away; however, I believed that Tonya knew in her heart that I was there with her in spirit. That was all that mattered to me. She knew that I loved her. A few days after that, her mother called to tell me that Tonya had passed. She left this earth on June 2, 2011. God had fixed it to where I was in a hotel room lying in bed from a flight layover when I received the news. Tonya had been in my life for six months, and I knew that God had put us together to encourage each other. Tonya showed me that no matter what was going on, to never stop praying and having faith. She continued to pray and love God in spite of what her body was going through. Despite the fact that she knew her time was near an end, she still loved God. She never expressed anger, bitterness, or disappointment towards Him. She was a soldier and was

*A Walking Miracle!*

faithful until the end. When her mother asked me to speak at the funeral, I initially said, *"No, I can't do that"* but then she said, *"Tonya would want you to."* I had never spoken at anyone's funeral before and I did not know if I could do it, but I spoke from the heart. I told everyone that Tonya had the strength of David and the faith of Job and Abraham.

After it was all over, I wondered *why* Tonya had to die and I was healed. I had so many mixed emotions and did not understand why she came into my life and left in six months. Although she was a blessing to me, and I'm so grateful to have known her and loved her, I was trying to understand and make sense of it all. She was so young with school-aged children and I was much older with adult children. I had lived much longer than Tonya and had done so much more. I suffered from survivor's guilt for a long time, but I discovered that sometimes God heals us in different ways and in response to the prayer of faith. Other times, He heals us and takes us to heaven, which Paul describes as far better. My question was why are some people healed when they pray with faith and others not? The

*Faith*

answer is, we don't know, and God doesn't always tell us. Who can know the mind of God? Tonya did not fail in her faith and her faith did not fail her. She was a wonderful example of trusting God in the most difficult of life's challenges. She will always be my sheroe of faith, and I was inspired by her unmovable trust and love for the Lord. She taught me to fight until the end.

    I remember what I wrote in my testimony that it's okay to cry. Big girls cry too! Therefore, I encourage people to cry whenever they feel like it; but it is equally important to laugh when you can, pray as much as you can, meditate, and most of all, believe. Tears are not a sign a weakness; they are a sign of strength. The Bible says that God takes our tears and stores them in His bottle (Psalm 56:8). The best person you can cry out to, is the Lord. Scream His name if you must. I did. I cried and called on Him to save my life and heal me, and He did. I had to figure out what would make me feel better and the only thing that could give me joy on the inside was the Lord. I knew I could run to Him and that He would hear me. I knew He was there with me and that He wasn't going to turn His back on me. I called my friend Sabrina Johnston, who had been diagnosed with breast cancer in 2006 and was now cancer free. She understood exactly what I was going through, the ups and the downs, the good days and bad days, the days of strength and the days of weaknesses. She understood it all because she had been there and done that. She allowed me to express my human emotions and she was right there to listen to me vent, cry, pray, or express whatever other feeling I was experiencing; and after I had released my frustrations, she let me know that I could make it. The key is not to grow weary or become frustrated. The sin is in not having faith. I had to be still, hold on to His Words, and give Him all the glory. I had to remember to remain positive, so whenever my emotions would change for the worse, I would shift them to focus on the positive. I was determined not to be afraid of tomorrow because His Word says that He will supply all my needs. He is my Shepherd. I shall not want anything (Psalm 23).

The Christian walk is a faith walk and it is not always easy. True faith is of the heart, not of the mind. As women,

*Faith*

we go through many things emotionally, psychologically, mentally and physically; and we still survive. We overcome and continue moving forward. God made us internally strong. Men could not handle half the things that we as women endure. Eleanor Roosevelt made the following statement that accurately describes how strong women are, and it is one of my personal favorites. *"A woman is like a tea bag. You never know how strong it is until it's in hot water."* What a true statement about women, and what we go through! As I consider the affliction that my body endured, and talk about the blessing of having faith, I cannot help but to identify with the woman who had the issue of blood that the Bible speaks of in Mathew Chapter nine. This woman knew beyond a shadow of a doubt that if she could just touch the hem of Jesus' garment, she would be healed. She did not doubt by saying to herself, "What if it doesn't work?" She had unwavering faith. She did not doubt in her heart. She had been bleeding for 12 years, had undergone many treatments, and yet she still suffered. She had seen many doctors and none could cure her. She was dying. Blood represents life.

*A Walking Miracle!*

She was losing blood each day from a slow hemorrhage, therefore she was losing life with each passing day. However, in spite of the many years, the many tears, the disappointments and wasted money, she never gave up. She had only heard about Jesus and His miracles, believed in her heart that He could heal her, and decided to find Him. She had faith in His miracle-working power. This woman was bold, but unassuming. She refused to let her prognosis be her death sentence. Many people tend to accept the prognosis given to them as their final analysis, but in spite of what you have been told, you still have God, the Master Physician and all He asks is that you trust Him by faith. By many standards, most would have given up and given in to their prognosis, but not this woman! She refused to let that sickness win the fight that she was in. Her strategic plan to press her way to Jesus was a decision of faith, and her persistence, boldness, and determination paid off. Her faith made her whole!

There is a power greater than yourself that operates upon your faith. The positive thoughts that you have about

*Faith*

your sickness mixed with faith creates the formula that will bring the healing. Faith is knowing regardless of what the outward conditions look like. Faith is trusting. Faith is acting. Faith is the evidence of things not seen with the natural eye, but knowing those things will manifest in the natural world. Faith honors God and yes, God honors faith. You must take your faith in God to a higher level and everything else will follow.

    God tests us, but He always brings us out of the test. He wants to see if we truly have faith in Him like we claim we do. Christians love to say they have faith until they really have to rely on it. My faith in God is unshaken because I know that He will never leave me nor forsake me. He never has and He never will. He moves by our acts of faith. Are you trusting God without seeing any evidence of deliverance in the natural realm? Faith is substance. Faith will bring the invisible substance into visible form. Got faith? We oftentimes do not understand why God allows certain things to happen in our lives and we get frustrated trying to figure it out. We wonder why we must struggle, we get mad with God

*A Walking Miracle!*

and feel the discouragement of worry, doubt and fear; but as His children, rooted and grounded in Christ, we continue to hold on to His promises because we know that weeping may endure for a night, but joy comes in the morning. When you have a strong foundation (Christ), nothing, no one, and no circumstance will shake your faith because you know that God sits on the throne and is still working things out for your good. When you are planted by the Lord, you will be able to withstand the violent storms of life without becoming uprooted. The faith that you have in God, in His power, and in His promises should supersede every negative situation that presents itself to you. Faith decides divine timing. How you deal with your test depends upon how fast He will bring you out. That is the time to pray and exercise the faith that you say you have. Faith is increased with spiritual vision. Sorrow looks back. Worry looks around, but faith looks up. I once read a quote on faith that I have added to my favorite quotes: *Faith is like a toothbrush, everyone should have one and use it daily, but they should not try to use someone*

*Faith*

else's. *Faith is not like gasoline which runs out as you use it, but like a muscle, which grows stronger as you exercise it.* It is time to walk your faith out. Stop just having faith and begin walking in faith.

When Satan comes knocking on your door, stop him at the porch and say, *"God, someone is at the door for you."* Let God answer. *Cast your burdens on the Lord and He will sustain you (Psalms 50:22).* If you don't pray and praise, Satan will move in and take up residency. Don't worry about anything, instead pray about everything. Tell God what you need and thank Him for all He has done thus far. Let Him direct you. He will take you to spiritual places that you never knew existed when you open yourself up to Hear from Him. Just as we need food and water for physical survival, we need Christ to live in us for spiritual survival. My faith has made me cancer free! My faith has made me whole. Bring all your issues to Jesus and let Him set you free in mind, body and spirit. I had to trust in the Lord with all my heart and soul in order to truly get healed. When you feel you cannot stand, lean on Him because He will direct your path. I put all my faith in Him when I felt that my

*A Walking Miracle!*

husband, family or friends did not understand how I was truly feeling on the inside. I had to trust God totally. At times, I felt like Dorothy from the Wizard of Oz. I had to follow the yellow brick road. I praise God because I am still standing on my faith.

When I think of the earthquake that hit Port-au-Prince Haiti in January 2010, I think of the faith that so many of the victims had in spite of that horrible tragedy. Thousands of people died that day. The town of Port-au-Prince was destroyed and people were left homeless. Some were trapped under buildings and a large number were badly injured. It was devastating to say the least. Sometimes faith is armed through traumatic situations such as that. For example, there were two women caught in the earthquake who were best friends. They were both terribly injured in the earthquake. A building fell on top of them and crushed the legs of both women. Both had their legs amputated. The amputations had to be performed immediately, but in the worst conditions, and without adequate medical equipment; but those two women were side by side strengthening each

*Faith*

other. They used one hand to hold the hand of the other and their other hand was lifted up praising and thanking the Lord. What faith these women had! We must hold on to our faith through the darkest times in our lives. Faith is so simple, but we make it complicated. We must hold on to faith when there seems to be no way out and when it looks as though there is no hope for the situation. We need faith even though we may have been diagnosed with a debilitating disease or condition. We must still hold on to our faith and trust the wisdom of God when babies die, when the economy is bad, when people are losing jobs, when parents pass on, and good people are suffering. We must trust the plan of God. When must see Him at work regardless of whatever comes our way. Cancer had my body, but it did not have my spirit. We must trust God knowing that He causes everything to work together for good, to them that love the Lord, to those who are the "called" according to His purpose (Romans 8:28). If you love God and you know that you have been called, then all things are working together for your good, not some things, but *all* things.

### Palm Tree Faith

When I was diagnosed with stage four breast cancer, I imagined myself in a category four hurricane planting my feet strong and stable like a palm tree whose roots grow deep into the ground. My body was the trunk of the palm tree swaying side to side with the wind, yet not breaking. My arms and hands were like leaves reaching up to God, believing in His Words. I could feel His love and favor. I knew this was not the end of my life, but the beginning of a new journey filled with joys and victories to be won. Just as the wind blows the leaves of the palm tree and the trunk of it, yet nothing breaks, you too must hold on to your faith in God, and do not break. Be grateful for all obstacles in your life and He will continue to strengthen you for this journey. We do not live by fear, but by faith.

Faith becomes noticeable everywhere. You can have faith at work, at home, and while you are doing recreational things. Your faith demonstrates that God is working in you. God will lead you to do things that you are only able to do through His Spirit, such as loving those who are not lovable, or who do not love you back. The Holy Spirit's guidance

*Faith*

will restrain you from doing things that your flesh wants to do, but should not do, such as treating people in the same negative way they have treated you. The peace of God has placed everything good in you so that you may do His will which is pleasing in His sight through Jesus Christ (Hebrews 3:20-21).

## Wavering Faith

It is natural for faith to waver from time to time. We are Christians, but we are still human, and every now and then, a strong Christian will waver in their faith; but the key is not to stay there. Remember God's promises in His Word. Remember all the good that He has done for you and the many blessings you have. This will bring your faith back to where it needs to be.

## Contentment

I have learned to be content. My testimony includes up and downs, a litany of doctor's appointments, anxiously waiting on test results, mammograms, x-rays, etc. I did not

*A Walking Miracle!*

always have a smile on my face or joy in my heart, and I don't always have a smile on my face now, but I do have joy in my heart. It is because I have learned contentment. Whatever state I am in, I have learned to be content in knowing that Jesus is aware of everything concerning me. Learning contentment requires belief in God's almighty power and faith that all things are possible through Him. God has the answer to all things; and because of my faith and belief, I know that "I can do all things through Christ who strengthens me" (Philippians 4:13). My faith and belief has given me spiritual muscles, and I am strong in the Lord! *"I have learned in whatever state I am in, to be content. I know both how to be abased, and I know how to abound: Everywhere and in all things I am instructed both to be full and to be hungry, both to abound and to suffer need. I can do all things through Christ which strengthens me (Philippians 4:11-13)!*

## POINTS TO PONDER

- In order to believe and know that God will heal you, you must have faith.

Without doubting and questioning, I had to trust that everything would be just fine because it always had been. Why do we sometimes have more faith in people and things than we do God?

There is a power greater than yourself that operates upon your faith. The positive thoughts that you have about your sickness mixed with faith creates the formula that will bring the healing speedily.

When Satan comes knocking on your door, stop him at the porch and say, *"God, someone is at the door for you."* Let God answer. *Cast your burdens on the Lord and He will sustain you (Psalms 50:22).*

# Chapter 3
# Your Attitude has Power

Webster's dictionary defines the word attitude as, *"a manner of acting, thinking, or feeling that shows one's disposition or opinion."* A person's attitude often dictates the circumstances that they find themselves in, and their attitude can also determine how they get out of circumstances. I have found that reading the Bible changes one's attitude as well as their disposition. By reading and absorbing God's Word, we learn how to look at life's trials through the eyes of the Lord and we are better able to handle them with the Word as our guide. We acquire wisdom, get spiritual revelation, and gain Godly insight through the Word. *For the Word of God is quick and powerful, and sharper than any two-edged sword, piercing even to the dividing asunder of soul and spirit, and of the joints and marrow, and is a discerner of the thoughts and*

*Your Attitude Has Power!*

*intents of the heart (Hebrews 4:12).* Being diagnosed with cancer, revealed just how strong I was. I have always been called the crybaby in my family, so on the outside, it seemed as though I was weak, but what matters is what's inside. I am a strong warrior on the inside. I am a fighter and a believer in God. Cancer showed me that!

Cancer starts from one cell then spreads to other cells. This disease is a quiet and mysterious one because a person can go on for years not knowing that cancer is in their body. Everyone has dormant cancer cells in their body, but when they are awakened, they can become deadly. They hide in the dark, then suddenly wake up and show their ugly head. If you are ever diagnosed with cancer, the first moments after hearing the news are those of disbelief, then your mind begins racing a thousand miles a minute. You will ask yourself, *Is this really happening to me?* then you will ask yourself, *Am I going to die?* After you have finally absorbed the news that

> "God has the power to do all things. He's the Master Physician. He doesn't need to "practice" because He gets it right the first time."

*A Walking Miracle!*

has just been told to you, you must imagine that you are in a war zone. You are on the battlefield and must understand that if you have any chance at all of beating your enemy (cancer), then you must enter this battle with a positive attitude in order to fight and win. Please understand that you can live a long and prosperous life after cancer. If you are going to win this war, you must think like a winner and a survivor. If you give in, it will take over and keep taking over until there is nothing more to take. I did not sign up to be in the war that I fought in. I was drafted to fight without any training. Knowing what I know now, I did not need any training. I had all I needed, which was my faith, courage, belief that I was going to beat this, and the Holy Spirit as my guide. I went straight to the top as a sergeant. God was my lieutenant. This was God's war. He was in charge and I followed His orders as a willing vessel.

    I had to learn that doing only what my oncologist told me to do was not enough. I had to work at healing myself. I have always exercised by walking and lifting weights. As a result of this, my body healed quickly after my lumpectomy surgery. However, my strength did not come from lifting weights. My strength came from lifting myself up in prayer and having faith in my God, who is the Master Physician who has never lost a patient. Walking helped me clear my mind and lower my stress level. Walking is an extremely valuable habit to alleviate stress. I stood on the promises of God's Word and held on to those promises. In my own battle with stage four cancer, my attitude kept my spirits high, although I had my sad moments at times. In order to beat cancer, I had to face this challenge with an attitude that I was going to do everything I needed to do in order to win this war. I was determined not to be a victim. I refused to cultivate a victim's *"why me, poor me"* mentality. I was determined to be victorious! To beat cancer, one cannot be passive and weak-minded no matter what the prognosis is. I highly respect doctors, but the truth is that they are not always right. They are called practitioners because they "practice" on patients. They are only *practicing* physicians. God is the all-knowing physician. He is still alive, still on the throne, and working miracles on behalf of

His children. I am a walking, talking, someone-you-can-touch, miracle!

### An Attitude of Faith

When faced with health issues, trials, hardships, divorces, financial problems and/or wayward children, we must understand that the devil will try to steal your faith. God tries our faith so we can try His faithfulness, but the devil tries to cause us to doubt God's Word so that our faith will weaken. He knows that you will win if you stay in faith and stand on God's promises. God is always near. Run to Him. There will be days that you will become a little discouraged, but the key is not to stay in that place. Do not give up even when you feel like you are falling and cannot get up. Reach out for His unchanging Hand. He will lift you up. Lean on Him. He will hold you up. I tell family and friends that if you ever see me walking and I am leaning to the side, that means I'm leaning on the Lord. He's guiding me and holding me up at the same time. Trust Him and believe in His Word. That's all. This applies to everyone

*Your Attitude Has Power!*

who has ever had a difficult test, trial, or major challenge in their lives. Everyone has a different cross to bear. Your cross may not be cancer. It may be another illness or maybe no illness at all. It could be financial, job-related, or family related. Whatever it is, I encourage you to trust in Him who has all the answers to your problems. Read, study, and meditate on His Word. You will learn what His promises are for your life and you can begin making declarations regarding the promises that He has spoken in His Word concerning you. Remember that your attitude will significantly impact how you will fight the war. Speaking from my experience and being a cancer warrior, I needed to be fed with prayer and hope, faith and courage. I left the war with a pink heart, a heart of thanksgiving, courage and love. I now have an honorable discharge!

> *"I left the war with a pink heart, a heart of thanksgiving, courage and love. I now have an honorable discharge!"*

When family and friends heard about my battle, they were eager to visit, call, or pray with me. Through their love

*A Walking Miracle!*

and support, I felt as though I was given powerful ammunition to fight: I had spiritual rifles, grenades, shotguns, handguns, magnum revolvers, and ak-47s. I was ready to fight and win! I knew I had an army of family, friends, and prayer warriors to back me up when I was on the front line of the battlefield. Although I was cultivating a positive attitude, there were days when I would become a little discouraged, but knowing that family and friends were rooting for me, my attitude became even more upbeat and positive. I never stayed discouraged for long. Most importantly, I knew that God was always with me and on my side fighting this battle with me. I knew that I was on the winner's side. God uses instances such as mine to get our attention in order to encourage us to trust and lean on Him. Whatever battle you are fighting right now, take your problem to the Lord and ask Him for the solution. *"Whatever you ask when you pray, believe that you will receive" (Mark 11:24).* Instead of complaining to God about how big your problem is, go to your problem and tell it how big your God is. It is under His control, not yours. He will not disappoint you. He is bringing you closer to Him through your adversities.

### Your Attitude is a Choice

Just as you choose the food you eat and the clothes you wear each day, you choose your attitude each day as well. A positive attitude is a choice. There is plenty to be thankful for. We can either choose to complain about things that do not go our way, or we can choose to be thankful for the blessings we do have. My point is that we all have daily choices to make. Being grateful is having a good attitude. As I look back over my life, I am grateful that God chose me. My attitude is still positive that I was diagnosed with cancer because it brought me closer to Him and strengthened my faith in His Word and in His healing power. My fight was a learning experience, yet a humbling one; but it was a test of my faith. My attitude gave me a different outlook and approach to life. God will put you right where He needs you to be, so don't let anyone steal your joy. Regardless of what the circumstances look like in the natural, know that God is working things out just for you. He can move heaven and hell just to bless you. When you look with your natural eyes only, you can be easily deceived by the devil, but when you listen to God's Holy Spirit when He speaks, you learn who is really in charge. He loves you and sometimes needs to purge you in order to take you higher in Him. My joy is in telling anyone who will listen to me for five minutes what God has done for me. If one chooses not to find the blessing in my story and take what they need from it, then that's on them. I just move on to the next person. God knows my heart. The main thing that was birthed from my journey is my story. I feel that it is my duty to share God's goodness with the world through my story of surviving stage four cancer. If you want to convince someone of what Christ will do for them, let them know what Christ has done for you. I have plenty to be thankful for. I am healthy. I am strong. I am living life to the fullest, and I am grateful that my **test** birthed my **test**imony. One of the most valuable gifts you can give a person is a piece of your heart and time by telling your testimony to them.

*Your Attitude Has Power!*

    In order to cultivate a good attitude, you must have a sound mind. If there is no peace in your life, there can be no peace in your mind; thus, there can be no positive thoughts. You cannot have a positive life and a negative mind. In order to have a positive life, you must have a positive mind. A positive outcome is the result of a positive mindset and this results in a positive attitude. It is written in His Word that God has given us a sound mind. *For God hath not given us the spirit of fear; but of power, and of love, and of a sound mind (2 Timothy 1:7-8).* When life becomes rocky and you ask God to smooth the road, go to His Word, because the answers are found there. Renew your mind daily with God's Word. No one ever said that this life would be easy. In fact, Jesus told us the contrary. He said that we would have tribulations. *In the world ye shall have tribulation: but be of good cheer; I have overcome the world (John 16:33b).* Everyone at some point in life will encounter their own tailor-made test. It is how you handle your tests that produces character, wisdom, and strength in you. You never know just how strong you are until you are severely tested.

*A Walking Miracle!*

Whatever is in you will come out when you are squeezed tight enough. If you squeeze a lemon, you will get lemon juice. If you squeeze an orange, you will get orange juice. When life puts the squeeze on you, then the true essence of who you are will come out. Although life squeezes you, you must still trust Him and praise Him. In order for a tree to come forth, a seed must die. In order for gold to be purified, it must go through the fire. To produce the wine, the grapes must be crushed, to produce the oil the olives must be pressed, to produce great strength in you, you must be purged through tests, trials, and difficulties. Everything comes with a cost. You must give up something in order to get something better. How would you respond if you or someone close to you were diagnosed with stage four breast cancer and was then told that the cancer was in the breasts, spine, hip, bones, and lymph nodes? Well, that was me, and that is exactly what I was told, but I am still here! I am still trusting God, I am still embracing my positive attitude, and I am cancer free!

## Questioning God

It is human nature to question God. I have heard people say that you should never question Him, but the truth is that we really do want answers. We want to know why certain things have happened. The only One who has all the answers about you is God, so why not ask Him questions. It is not His desire to have us ignorant of things concerning us. It is in His nature to communicate with us and bring us into knowledge and revelation about ourselves. I did ask God the question, *"Why did this happen to me? What did I do wrong?"* He sometimes answers, and He sometimes doesn't. If He decides not to answer you right away, then He will bring you to a place of peace, which will enable you to handle the situation at some point later on. You will eventually get the revelation - or you may not; but God is so faithful that He will not allow you to focus so much on the "why" but He will give you the courage and strength to overcome your situation with Him by your side. I got to a place that I shifted from *"Lord, why me?"* to *"Lord, why not me?"*

*A Walking Miracle!*

### An Attitude of Gratitude

In spite of my circumstances, I learned early in my fight, that there was always someone in a far worse condition than I was. I thought that being diagnosed with stage four breast cancer was one of the worse things that could happen to anyone, but then I saw others with cancer who were receiving chemotherapy and were too weak to even sit up. I saw some patients who had been badly burned from radiation. I saw others who were on oxygen tanks because the cancer had taken over their lungs and they couldn't breathe on their own. There were others who were completely bald from the chemotherapy. Unfortunately, I also met people while on this journey who lost their fight with cancer. My heart bled for those people and was filled with compassion for all of them. I thought that my situation was bad, but God allowed me to see that it was not as bad as I initially thought it was. It could have been much worse. Seeing those precious people put life in perspective for me. It made me more grateful for my "light affliction." *For our light affliction, which is but for a moment, works for us a far more exceeding and eternal weight of glory (2 Corinthians*

*Your Attitude Has Power!*

*4:17-18)*. Although I was diagnosed with cancer and was told that it had spread to various places in my body, I did not have any chemotherapy or radiation; nor did I have a mastectomy. My breasts are still intact. It is also important to confess that I never had a day of weakness and I never got sick during this journey.

To some, being told that they have cancer is equivalent to being given a death sentence. Life is really put in perspective when this news is given. For me, it revealed how precious life really is. Every day that I woke up and was able to see the sunrise and set, made me thankful. A cancer diagnosis affects each person differently. Some people choose to become and remain bitter, thinking that life has treated them unfairly. They blame God and become angry with Him. Unfortunately, some of those people die with that same mindset. Their negative attitude feeds their cancer. Still, there are others, who were diagnosed with cancer, but died. They should not have. Some of them did not fight. They chose to give up. They allowed stress to take residence in their mind. Cancer feeds on stress and causes it to spread rapidly. They were never able to rise above the diagnosis. Their test was designed to make them stronger, but they looked at it as a reason to weaken them. This is not to say in no way, that everyone who died from cancer didn't fight. This is to say that there is a segment of people who gave up when they could have fought a little harder. For others, cancer forces them to do the things they have always wanted to do, but had been putting those things off. My diagnoses made me realize that each day is precious and should be lived to the fullest. It essentially made me a better person in many ways. I had dreams that I made come true. Writing this book has become a dream come true. I had never thought of writing a book before my diagnosis, but it is my duty to tell my story and what better way to share it with the masses than putting it in a book? This is my legacy to my children, my grandchildren and their children. My diagnosis also forced me to take a much-needed trip to clear my head. After my diagnosis, my husband and I went to Jamaica for three days and two nights. If it were not for the diagnosis, I do not think I would have gotten on a water ski. All my life, I have been afraid of the water - especially the ocean. The only

*Your Attitude Has Power!*

thing I do with water is wash with it and drink it in an eight-ounce glass. With a life jacket on my back, and arms tightly around the driver, I felt safe, just as I feel now with God's arms wrapped around me, watching over me, and cheering me on. Cancer motivated me to do something I probably never would have done.

    My goal is to encourage patients that when they hear the word cancer, it does not mean imminent death. It does not mean toe tag. In spite of your diagnoses, as long as you awaken each day and are able to see the sun, then live with an attitude of gratitude. You are in God's hands. He is shielding you from the attack of the enemy. Remember this is God's war. Let Him fight it through you.

### From Winter to Springtime

    Sometimes I felt like I was in the dead of winter with no shelter and no weather coat. At times, I felt that I had no hope, but God knew me better than I knew myself. He was confident in my tenacity and in my ability to rise above my test. He is my strength. He trusted me in my battle with

*A Walking Miracle!*

Satan. I was in a blizzard, but my faith brought me into springtime. The trees sprouted green leaves and flowers began to blossom. The sun began to shine as my winter started to disappear; so when the winter of your life brings a blizzard, cover up, put on your winter boots, and continue to move and believe that springtime is just around the corner.

**Bag Lady**

After I screamed and cried when the doctor initially said I needed a mastectomy, chemotherapy, *and* radiation, a peace eventually came over me. That was the outer me that screamed and cried, but the inner me showed up, the mighty warrior. I then held my shoulders back, my head up, and said, *"This my bag."* In other words, people have all kinds of bags that they pick up along the journey of life, and this diagnosis was just one of my bags. As a flight attendant for almost 40 years (as of this writing), I can certainly relate to baggage. My job requires me to carry bags all over the world. Our perspective about things that happen to us in life comes from what we have experienced, been exposed to, and what we have seen. I am seeing things from the perspective of being a flight attendant and having carried bags all over the world for so many years. However, this new bag was very different, but the same in many ways. It was different because it was a much heavier bag with difficult contents, but the same, because although I have to carry it, I am still helping others to carry theirs. I had two options. I could carry this bag and have a good attitude about it, or drag this bag and allow it to weigh me down. I chose the first option. My attitude changed and I was determined to fight, and fight hard until I got rid of this heavy bag. I thought of James Brown's song 'Papa's got a brand new Bag', well... Trisha's got a brand new bag too! Patty Labelle sings the song called, 'I've got a new Attitude'. In the song, she also says that she's got a new dress and a new hairdo too. For me, I've got a new attitude to go with my new bag. I believe in many ways that this is the reason I was "blessed" to have taken this journey - to help others carry their bags after receiving their diagnosis. Yes, I say "blessed" because so much good has come out of my story. I could have chosen to have a different

*A Walking Miracle!*

attitude and look at what seemed to be negative and devastating, but instead, I chose to look at the positive side of it. Today I am helping other cancer patients to carry their bags. I talk to them about the benefits of having a good attitude. Tom Hanks in the movie 'Forest Gump' pinned a famous line, which resonates so true about life: *"Life is like a box of chocolates; you never know what you are going to get."* Well, I will say amen to that! Who would have ever thought that being a flight attendant would help me to carry this heavy bag and to teach other people how to carry whatever heavy burden life has placed on them?

### Change and Choices

God gave me a choice. Life is about choices and He gives us free-will and self-choice. I *chose* a good attitude, which helped to renew my body. I believe that God was proud of my decision. My mind, soul and spirit were strengthened as I leaned on Him for guidance and help. My daily prayer was for God to prepare me for whatever comes my way. My prayer is still the same and I also ask Him to minister to my spirit by way of His Holy Spirit.

*Your Attitude Has Power!*

Where there is pain, He will give His peace and mercy. Where there is self-doubt, He will give His confidence. Where there is weariness, He will give His strength and His grace.

We cannot always change other people's ways or attitudes, but we can show them the benefits of embracing a good attitude by way of example. The only person we can truly change is ourselves. By our goodness, patience, calmness and smiles, they will see the peace that goes along with being positive, and if they want to change, they will change. That is the kind of impact that we can have on others. We can be the change agent by being the change. Always remember that you can only change yourself with God by your side. When you take the first step, He will take the next one for you.

For a person who has lived their life being negative, it will not be easy to suddenly change, but with effort, a change in attitude can be made. When a cancer diagnosis is made, it is critical that we keep our thoughts positive. Negative thinking brings on negative actions and negative actions bring negative circumstances. With God's help, through His Holy Spirit, a positive attitude can be birthed on the inside. Just allow the Holy Spirit to speak to you from within. Life is too short to waste time on negative thinking. Focus on the good things God has done and is still doing in your life. It is important to read your Bible and strive to be happy and to have a positive outlook no matter what life has brought your way. *"Rejoice always, pray without ceasing in everything, and give thanks, for this is the will of God in Christ Jesus concerning you" (1 Thessalonians 5:16-18).*

    I discovered that each person's attitude is much different from the next person. The circumstances can be the exact same, but the reactions are much different and will vary from person to person. As I said before, our circumstances and experiences in life determine how we react to things. If you are generally a positive person, then you will see some good that will be birthed from the situation. If you are a negative person, then you will see everything about your diagnosis from a negative perspective. When you blame others for your unhappiness, illness, or loss

*Your Attitude Has Power!*

of a loved one, you are giving your power to the wrong things. You can direct your mind to have peace, love, and faith. You must trust in the Lord with all your heart and lean not on your understanding.

If you are a football lover, then think about it like this: your body is the football team. Every part has a special position to play: the quarterback, the linebacker, running back, wide receiver, and the kicker. Your objective is to make the final touchdown in order to win the game. In order to make that touchdown and take your health back, you must carry the football all the way to the end zone - blocking.... dodging... and running faster than the opposing team. Listen to your coaches. They are your doctors, which include your oncologist, surgeon, nutritionals, therapist, technicians, and all other medical staff who have your best interest at heart. Stay in the game by eliminating certain foods and starting your exercise regimen. You must keep a positive attitude throughout all of this and you must do your part. No negotiations! You must take charge of your life, starting with your health. You must refuse to lose. Giving up is not an option. You must fight for your life. Pray always.

### New Attitude

I was knocked down but I was not knocked out. To be a winner, you must face your adversity head on, grab it and tackle it. When I became afraid, I continued to pray until I grew stronger. When I became afraid, I took deep breaths and focused on my breathing. I would also take long walks to clear my mind in order to gain clarity. The sunshine and oxygen assists with mental clarity and is good for physical health as well. I discovered that it is also imperative to listen to your body. In other words, when you become tired, take time to rest. Also, take the time to laugh, smile, and have fun. Laugher is good medication for cancer. When you smile, your digestion improves. When you chuckle, your burdens are lightened. When you laugh, your life is lengthened, because laughter is the great secret to a long life. You only live once. Life is short, so savor the moments! If you are in a battle, be in it to win it and finish first!

*Your Attitude Has Power!*

Praising God in spite of your circumstances is a powerful weapon that weakens the enemy. Sometimes it may seem like the answer is taking too long, but praising and thanking God will strengthen your faith and increase your patience. Doing this gave me the strength to face each day, and I was ready for what each day contained. When it seems that life has thrown you a curve ball, look for the lesson in the situation and keep in mind that every test is designed to strengthen your character, increase your faith and bring you closer to God. When I plant my flower garden, not only will flowers grow, but sometimes weeds will grow in the same garden, so it is my job to remove the weeds. Just as you remove the weeds from your flower garden, you have to weed out self-doubt and negative thinking and replace them with confidence and a good attitude. Your mind is your flower garden. Do not worry about yesterday. It is dead and gone. You must focus on the *now*. We must learn to live in the present moment. Do not steal from the present by worrying about the future or crying over the past. Live to the fullest today. If you do, then your future will be very bright.

*A Walking Miracle!*

## Thanksgiving Fast

Reflecting over my life and all that had transpired in the previous months made me deeply thankful for the grace and mercy that God has bestowed upon me. I decided to go on a 21-day Thanksgiving fast. The purpose of the fast was to give thanks and not to complain about anything for 21 days - nothing! No, it was not during the Thanksgiving holiday, but it was still a time of thanksgiving for me. The objective of my fast was to wake up each day and be thankful for everything - good and bad. Oftentimes, we do not realize that we are complaining, especially when it comes to those things that are perfectly justifiable to complain about. These include things such as long lines in the grocery store, rush hour traffic, the TSA lines at the airport, the cost of gas, etc., but during my 21-day fast, the focus was to complain about absolutely nothing. It is amazing that we do not realize how much we complain about things when we are not cognizant of it, but since I was diligently watching my thoughts, I recognized when a complaint would try to come up, and I immediately dismissed it. It was an experience. When the fast was over, I

*Your Attitude Has Power!*

had become a better person as I continued to embrace the same focus I had during the fast. My daily focus was to remember the days of blessings and forget the days of troubles. I always keep in mind that nothing is random and that everything has purpose. I have found that when we start giving thanks to God for *all* things, we feel connected to God all throughout the day. It is in the presence of the Lord that a refreshing takes place. The Lord desires to refresh and restore His children, but in order to receive restoration and a refreshing, you must be in place to receive it. Restoration happens in the presence of the Lord. In His presence is the fullness of joy! In the Word of God and in the presence of the Lord is where faith is built up and joy is given. When you stay in faith and stay in the Word, you become stronger, wiser and ready to face whatever test that life brings your way. Everyone in this life must go through a trying time, but God has given each of us the internal strength to endure and overcome every test and trial. This is the only way that we can be taken to another level. God desires to bless each of His children, but the blessings do not come easy. We must

*A Walking Miracle!*

pass our tests. After that, we are blessed beyond measure. God is the Giver of all good things and He will give you your heart's desires; but we must never let the abundance of God's gifts cause us to forget the Giver. We must desire God the Giver more than we desire His gifts. Only God can turn a mess into a message, a test into a testimony, a trial into a triumph, and a victim into a victory! In this life, we have both sunshine and rain. Rainy days may not be a favorite, but like all others days, they offer something positive, and since all days are God's days, a blessing can always be found in a storm cloud. Keep that in mind the next time you go through a storm in life.

### POINTS TO PONDER

- We acquire wisdom, get spiritual revelation and gain Godly insight through the Word.

- God tries our faith so we can try His faithfulness, but the devil tries to cause us to doubt God's Word so that our faith will weaken.

- There is plenty to be thankful for. We can either choose to complain about things that do not go our way, or we can choose to be thankful for the blessings we do have.

Only God can turn a mess into message, a test into a testimony, a trial into a triumph, and a victim into a victory!

# Faithful Family
# Chapter 4

As I look back over my life as a child, teenager, and young adult, I can honestly say that I had a happy life growing up. I was born and raised in Miami, Florida and my mother gave birth to me in the home that she and my father were living in as a married couple. During those times, the doctor would come to the home to deliver babies. I attended elementary to high school in Miami and had many friends. The bedroom I was born in was the same room I shared with my sister growing up. I have wonderful memories being raised by my parents. My late mother was the funniest person I've ever met. She had such a sense of humor and was extremely energetic. She would come outside and join in the baseball games when we would be outside playing with our friends. She was the only adult in the game filled with children. She would also sneak outside at night and scratch on the windows to scare my sister and I when we were in our bedroom. With my mother's sense of humor, our home was filled with laughter growing up. She kept the family radiant and full of joy. My mother deposited in me that same sense of humor. She also

*Faithful Family*

taught us that it was all right to laugh at yourself. In addition to humor, both my parents taught me the importance of respect for others, hard work, discipline, and self-confidence. My father was more laid back than my mother, although he did and said funny things at times too. I think my mother's personality rubbed off on him and every now and then, he would become a comic, but certainly not as much as my mother.

The most important life lesson that I learned from my parents was to respect yourself and others. We were taught to always be kind to people when we could, and my mother demonstrated that value that she taught us. She worked at our local elementary school as a part-time cafeteria assistant and was kind to all of the children. I enjoyed having my mother working in the same school I attended. It gave me a sense of security knowing that if anything went wrong, mommy was close by. Her "be kind to all" advice was shown in her as I think back on a student in the school who had a severe behavior problem. He was rude, insolent, and very disrespectful. My mother was the only person who could control his temper. She showed him love, kindness, and patience. My sisters and I could not understand why our

*A Walking Miracle!*

mother would take out so much of her time with that disrespectful, undisciplined little boy. He was just plain bad!

But I saw that around my mother, he melted. She had a positive impact on this student, and I could see the difference she made in his life. I don't think he had gotten attention or was shown love at home, and it was being expressed in negative ways. I think my mother filled the void that he had from not having anyone to love him. My mother would stress to us to be kind to others. I remember her constantly telling us that if we are kind and treat people with respect, then life's trials will probably work itself out; but if we are not kind to others, then life may not have any meaning.

That teaching has remained with me all of my life and I have seen the benefits of being kind to others. Kindness is a boomerang that comes back in a very positive way. As much as I can, I try to give a kind word to those I meet, even if it's just a smile. Because of that personality trait that was ingrained in me, so many people bent over backwards to be there for me through my diagnosis. While experiencing the process of having breast cancer and all that it entails, I always kept in my mind that no matter what is going on, my attitude and kindness can make it better. Therefore, it was not in me to become bitter. Of course, I had my discouraging days, but I never got bitter. In fact, I got better. I tried to laugh as much as I could, and the spirit of my mother's sense of humor sustained me in days when I would think on her. In many ways, I feel that my mother contributed to my healing through her spirit that remains with me. Both my parents have since passed on, but I'm thankful for the values they placed inside their children.

### My Husband, My Soulmate, My Friend

My husband, who is my closest friend was with me through this journey from beginning to end. He never left my side. He was there when I was first diagnosed. He accompanied me to all of my treatments, and was by my side during my surgery. His presence and devotion was, and still is a blessing for which I am thankful. My children on the other hand had a different perspective of how they viewed my situation. I only have two sons and they were 22 and 27

*A Walking Miracle!*

at the time. The day that I was first diagnosed, I went home and told both of my sons at the same time. I downplayed the diagnoses and told them that I was going to be just fine. I explained that I would have a lumpectomy and after that, I would be okay. From their expressions, they seemed to be fine. I am assuming that when they saw how calm and assured I was, they reacted off of me. When we overact to things, the situation can get worse, but when we exercise calmness as we are giving bad news, the situation can remain calm.

When I was informed that I was at a stage four and not a stage two as originally stated, I did not know how to tell my sons, so I arranged a meeting with them, my husband, and myself for the psychologist to break the news to them. We all rode together to meet the psychologist. My sons did not ask why we were going to meet the psychologist, but they willingly came along. At the meeting, she explained to them that I had stage four cancer and that it had spread to various places in my body, but she assured them that I would be okay. She then asked them what they

*Faithful Family*

were thinking about after hearing the news. Patrick said, *"My mom is very strong."* He did express that he wished I would have told them instead of bringing them there to be told by someone else. When she asked Chris what he was thinking, he only said, *"She's strong."* She could not pull anything else out of him. Patrick, my oldest son is more like me. He will talk and ask questions, but Chris, the youngest is more like his father. He internalizes things. Reactions to news like that are different for different people and we cannot expect everyone to respond the same way. Sometimes they become angry with the patient because they fear that the person is going to die, so they displace their aggression, hurt, and fear. Throughout the process, family may even hurt you with their attitudes and dispositions, but we must understand that at the root of their anger is fear and hurt. A week or so after the meeting with the therapist, I came home and explained to my oldest son Patrick that I would be having a mastectomy instead of the lumpectomy. My other son was not home at the time. He then called his brother, my youngest son and gave him the news. I am not sure how he

*A Walking Miracle!*

processed that news, but he was so upset that he would not come home. He called me crying and saying that he did not want to see me. I begged him to come home, but he refused. Finally, around midnight, he came home. He was scared of what my outcome would be. I believe that he thought that I was soon to die. When he entered my bedroom, my first reaction was to hold my child in my arms and rock him like I did when he was a baby, but he was a 6'3 grown man, so I had him sit on a stool next to my bed and lay his head in my lap. I kept trying to reassure him that I was going to be fine. He finally cried himself to sleep. We must closely watch those who hold things inside and do not outwardly show their emotions. They are the ones most inclined to explode from holding so much inside. My oldest son is a bit stronger. He even had his coworkers pray for me.

My attitude remained positive throughout all of this. When people would call me or come by to visit, I would declare that I knew that I was healed and that I was going to be just fine. For some reason, Patrick, the oldest, did not like me talking about my situation so much. He told a friend of

*Faithful Family*

mine that he felt that I wanted people to feel sorry for me. I was oblivious to the fact that his anger was increasing every time he heard me talking about my situation. When some people are diagnosed, they do not tell anyone. They keep their secret hidden and there is no outlet of expression for them. Talking about it is a healthy and healing practice. It was a form of therapy for me and every time I spoke affirmatively about my healing, I was releasing seeds that would return a healing harvest back to me, but my son did not see it that way. He felt that I wanted attention and/or for people to feel sorry for me. When I was told that he made that statement, I was deeply hurt. I didn't say anything to him right away, but decided to take him to lunch to talk about it. Sitting across from him, I could see the anger on his face. I did not understand why he was so upset, but I could see it all over him. It was almost a look of hatred that I saw. While at lunch, I asked him why would he tell people that I wanted them to feel sorry for me. I had never cried to anyone, never complained, never asked "why me?" to anyone, or exhibited emotions or words that I was feeling

*A Walking Miracle!*

sorry for myself. In spite of my diagnosis, my conversations were always upbeat and positive. I always spoke matter-of-factly about my healing, so what was my son thinking about me? After asking him the question, he said, *"If you are healed like you say you are, then why do you keep talking about it?"* I tried to explain to him that this was what God wanted me to do. He wanted me to be a testimony to people. My eyes filled with tears and I started to cry, then he said, *"Look at you, you use to be so strong. You're not strong anymore."* I started to reach into my purse to pay and then leave, but he jumped up and said, *"You don't have to leave, I'll leave!"* He left me right there in tears. People in the restaurant where watching us and probably thought that I was a "cougar" who had just had a fight with my younger boyfriend. I sat there for about ten more minutes to regain my composure, then I left. I sat in my car and cried until I couldn't cry anymore, then I drove off.

I had to understand that Patrick was not in the same spiritual place that I was. He had not been touched by death and did not have the level of intimacy with God as I had. Even though it hurt me, I understood that the devil was

*Faithful Family*

coming at me through my child, but I was not going to let it work. The devil was angry that I was so positive about my situation and he expressed his anger through my child. Life is about how we respond to offenses, tests, trials, tribulations and hardships when they are presented to us. I knew that my outlook would determine my outcome and I continued to speak blessings and healing over my life, in spite of what my son or anyone else thought.

> *"I knew that my outlook would determine my outcome and I continued to speak blessings and healing over my life, in spite of what my son or anyone else thought."*

When God made women, He made us special, with a formula much different from that of men. We are physically inferior to men, but emotionally, mentally, and psychologically, we are stronger. We can carry the weight of the world on our shoulders, yet still be compassionate enough to give comfort and nurturing. We have the inner strength to endure childbirth and withstand rejection that comes from the men in our lives, including our children. We have the maternal sensitivity to love our children under any situation, even when they hurt us. A woman's beauty is not determined by wearing her hair long, short, or bald; nor is it in the fashion she puts on, or the figure she carries. It is not in her stature as short, tall, fat or slim; but her beauty is in her eyes, her heart, and the love that is in her spirit. It is in the faith she has in her God. Essentially, the beauty of a woman does not come from the outer. The beauty in me causes me to love my children no matter what.

It has been said, but definitely bears repeating, that my husband was there for me from the very beginning of my diagnosis until the day that I was pronounced as cancer free. I've always known that my husband was a good man, a loving husband, a provider, and an excellent father; but as the years progressed, he proved himself to also be a wonderful grandfather, uncle, and friend; but it wasn't until my cancer diagnoses that I recognized just how much of a jewel he really is. He held me, encouraged me, cried with me, and even made me laugh. He never left my side. He was right there with me late at night when I would cry out for my mother, who died many years ago. He was right there when I would cry out to the Lord asking Him to heal me. There were times when I would wake up to find him watching me sleep. He refused to stay away from even one of my doctor's appointments and was there for every PET scan, MRI, and bone scan, except one. He only missed that one because my friend Gwen begged him to let her take me to the appointment instead of him, and he finally gave in.

### For Better or for Worse

My husband and I have known each other since the 7th grade. We began dating in the 9$^{th}$ grade. Through young adolescent dating, we broke up, reunited, broke up again, and eventually reunited for one last time. True love will always find its way back home. My husband calls me three times a day to see if everything with me is fine. When there are days that I may not be feeling well, he's willing to stay home from work to be with me, even if it's only a cold that I have. God gave me the right man, and I'm deeply grateful for that. My husband is a gift from God and I'm thankful that I am married to my true, God-given soulmate. In many ways, my husband reminds me of my daddy. When my mother was bedridden, my daddy retired so that he could be home to make sure that the round-the-clock nurses were taking good care of her. In like manner, my husband was right there as well, watching, protecting, and comforting me. He has been to me, what my father was to my mother. Throughout my process of being diagnosed with breast cancer and all that I underwent in between, my husband never caused me one day of stress. Stress and cancer do not mix. I have heard the stories of those who, although diagnosed with cancer, also had to deal with inconsiderate and verbally abusive mates, mounting bills, ungrateful children and a range of different issues that gave them no peace, but more stress. Stress feeds cancer, so a patient must try to remain peaceful and calm throughout the process of getting treatment. A stress-free life plays a critical role in the process. With my husband by my side, I never had to worry about any stress. Over time, I have come to realize that the most precious things in life are not material possessions. That's just "stuff". People who love me, stuck by me, and encouraged me are what are most valuable to me. That is what is truly precious.

## My Five Heartbeats

My parents had four girls and they raised us to be very close. It was instilled in us that family comes first and when I was diagnosed with cancer, the Barnes girls were in shock, but were ready to unite together and do whatever needed to be done for me. Even though each of them had a different reaction to the news, they were still ready to be by my side and help alleviate any unnecessary burden.

My sister Lonzie, who we call Mancy, lives in Colorado and is a hospice Minister. In her experience, she has seen many patients suffer with cancer. Her job is to help prepare them for their transition. She called everyday to pray with me and to find out how I was feeling. I would always say, "I'm fine". She did not come down to Miami when I had the surgery, and I couldn't understand that. I knew she loved me, and was genuinely concerned about me. Since our mother has passed on, I look up to her as my mother although she is my big sister. My love, respect and admiration for her exceeds just sibling love. After all, she changed my diapers and cared for me to help my mother out at times. I thought for sure that she would be there for my surgery. I longed for her presence, but I tried not to dwell on it. After the surgery, however, she came down, and went with me to my doctor's appointment. She stayed while I received my treatments. She thanked all the doctors, nurses and technicians for taking care of me and she even took pictures. I was filled with joy to have my big sister right there by my side.

Stella, my second oldest sister who lives in Valdosta, Georgia also called regularly to check on me, but she never came down, and I wondered why. Again, I knew that she loved me, but I wanted her there. When I asked her why she didn't come, she said she didn't know. She felt that deep down inside I would be fine, but I wanted her by my side. I had no doubt in my mind that all my sisters loved me deeply and I understand that reactions from family members are different. Just because they may not have been there physically, did not mean they were not there in spirit and their love for me is not diminished because of it.

*Faithful Family*

Yvonne, the youngest sister was there from the very beginning. With her by my side, I did not have to think about anything other than getting well. She wrote down all of my appointments, then would call to remind me of days and times. If for whatever reason, she could not accompany me, she made sure that there was always a woman there who came with me. I will never forget the day that she told me to get in the shower and cry, scream, pray, ask God to forgive me of my sins, then ask Him to heal me. I did it. I cried out to Lord and He heard me. She took me right back to the ABC concept. **A**ccept Jesus, **B**elieve in Him, and **C**onfess your sins. Many people do not realize that confessing their sins plays a major role in healing. Unconfessed sins is what sometimes allows sickness and disease to linger, but when we confess our sins, and release them to God, they have no license to hang around and manifest in the body in the form of disease. Confession of sins opens the door to healing and makes sickness and disease leave out of that same door. Thank you for that gift Yvonne. Telling me to do that not only changed my life, but saved my life!

Karen and I have been in each other's lives since first grade. They cannot be called "best friends" because they are my sisters. I gave Karen her own nickname especially from me called Curlen. When her mother would hear me call her

*A Walking Miracle!*

that, she would say, *"Her name is Karen. Repeat after me, K a r e n"*, but I would say, *"C u r l e n"*. That was my special name for her and to this very day, I am the only one who calls her that. We do not speak very often, but when we do, it's as though we never lost a day. After my diagnosis, we spoke regularly. She surprised me in December 2008, at my home with a small live Christmas tree decorated all in purple. She knew that purple was my favorite color, so she wanted me to feel special and loved, and I was. It's not always the big things in life that makes us smile, it's the little things that mean the most. I will never forget that special Christmas in 2008 when my sister showed up on my doorstep with a beautiful purple Christmas tree. Curlen, I love you sis!

    Adria Harrison-Wiley is also not a blood relative, but she is definitely one of my sisters. We lived in the same neighborhood, and attended the same elementary school. If I cried in class for something, Adria would cry too. When the teacher would ask her why she was crying, she would say, *"I am crying because Tricia's crying."* We still cry together to this very day. If one of us are going through a rough time, we both are going through. That is how special our bond is. Adria is so much more than just a friend. We are just as close as my blood sisters, and my biological sisters consider her as their sister too. Thank you Adria for being there when I needed you as I was battling cancer. I love you dearly sis!

**Vitamin "F"**

Did you know that having friends is good for your health? Dr. Oz calls them vitamin F. He counts the benefits of friends as essential to our well-being. Research shows that people in a strong social circle have less risk of depression and terminal strokes. Having a variety of friends brings out a different part of me because some seem to understand me better than I understand myself. I am happy that I have a stock of vitamin F! It stops stress and in my darkest moments, it decreases the chance of a heart attack or a stroke by 50%. This is why I value and keep in touch with my friends; so we can laugh at new and old experiences and pray for each other in tough times. When I was a little girl, my concept of a best friend was only one person, but when I was diagnosed with cancer, I realized that I had many "best" friends. They were all the best at various things in their own ways. If you ask Him, God will show you the "best" of many friends. For me, there is one friend for every day of the week, and then some leftover. One friend is there to hear me vent when I'm going through challenges with my husband. Another friend is perfect for when I'm having challenges

*A Walking Miracle!*

with family members. Another was always there when I was giving birth, and then there in the bleachers with me cheering my children on with excitement and delight during little league games. Still, there are some who are right there when it's time to shop, and then those who are there when I need to share, heal, hurt, joke, or just be who I am. One friend cries with me when I cry, and there are a few friends who meet my spiritual needs saying, *"If we pray together and believe that we are bigger than cancer, then we should never give up or give in."* Another has a shoe fetish like me, while another has a love for movies, another is right there when I'm confused about life and still another is there to help me understand things and keep me calm. We cannot choose our family members, but we can choose good friends. Things change in life just like the weather, jobs, and locations. Friends may come and go, but if you are blessed, your real friends stay throughout your entire life.

I am blessed to have several friends who I can go to for whatever it is that I need. They each entered my life in different seasons and have remained with me along this journey. I have childhood friends from elementary school going all the way back to first grade, some from high school,

*Faithful Family*

and a few from college. I have some friends from past jobs and others who I have met at various places. I consider family members as friends as well. My friends and family have made me the woman I am today. I survive because I have a circle of friends who had and still have my back. They are a phenomenal support system for me. They had faith in my healing when my own faith was slacking. They knew some good prayers to pray in order to change things. They kept me focused and for that, I'm grateful. Through them, God was with me and showed me His love.

There will be times in everyone's life when trials, tribulations, hardships, difficulties, or some sort of challenge will come knocking on the door. Oftentimes these tests blindside us and we have no power over them. The power we do have however, is the ability to trust that God has divine purposes for these tailor-made situations. We must fulfill whatever God has placed in our lives and not try to figure things out on our own, because we will not understand the mystery behind what God does. All we know is that He is working things out for our good. We must simply fulfill the

*A Walking Miracle!*

task that He has assigned because He knows what He has planned for our lives. Stay strong and keep looking forward. Never look back.

The great women in the Bible did not start as great. They each went through something traumatic, heartbreaking, or devastating before they could be perceived as great. Mary Magdalene, Ruth, Naomi, the woman with the issue of blood, Hannah, Esther, Rachel and Leah all had to go through something challenging. Mary Magdalene was a loose woman, but after her encounter with Jesus, she was His closest follower. Esther was an orphan being raised by her older cousin Mordecai, but God had a plan for her life, and by the time God's plan was fulfilled, she had married one of the wealthiest men in the land, the King. Each phenomenal woman in the Bible had a story to tell, but their faith and trust in God allowed them to overcome their tests. A woman sometimes has to look closely at her own life and consider her glory as well as her imperfections. After my cancer diagnosis, I felt as though I was a messed up failure. It seemed that one thing after another was happening to me.

*Faithful Family*

## Qualities of Friends

Good friends are faithful as well as honest with you, they respect you for who you are and what you stand for; they keep you in the loop, encourage you when needed, and express that they need you as a friend too. True friends will stand by you, and will stand with you. If a friend or so-called friend does not have these qualities, you may question their true friendship. These are the ones you may have to let go somewhere down the line. Be able to walk away. It does not mean that you are mean or not loving, or do not care, but the fact remains that everyone is not your friend. All you can do is pray for them and wish them the best. Pray for guidance because God will show you who your true friends are. You always have a friend in Him. He is the Friend that sticks closer than a brother (Proverbs 18:24).

Friendship is one of God's greatest gifts. He is the most loyal and true Friend. At those times when there is no friend around, you can always depend on God to be a constant friend. He's dependable, always available for you, and will not talk about you behind your back. Sometimes our friends disappoint us by not being there when we need them the most, not calling, even talking behind our backs. When you depend on a friend, you have to realize they can be replaced. Friends are wonderful to talk to and it is therapeutic to have someone to express feelings, but when there is no friend around, you can pray and cry out loud to your constant Friend, and He will hear your voice. He's always there. Go to Him to talk. He is present when no one else is. Remember when you need Him, it doesn't matter what time it is, you can depend on His presence.

## A Mirror In God's Hand
### By Paula Fox

I want to be a mirror Lord, a reflection of your grace;
to shine your light for all to see in every darkened place.
I want to be transfigured Lord, so your image others see;
and be closer to your likeness, and the light you've given me.
I have no light source of my own, but when I look at you,
the radiance of your glory shines in all I say and do.
I could stand to use some polish; I've been
cracked and broken too;
but it's not myself that matters, it's the light that
comes from you.
Though I have some imperfection,

I'm still useful in your sight,
and in your hand I know, that you will angle me just right.
So that when you shine on me, it reflects on others too,
And as it pleases you to use me Lord, to light
my world for You!

## POINTS TO PONDER

- Essentially, the beauty of a woman does not come from the outer. The beauty in me causes me to love my children no matter what.

- Stress feeds cancer, so a patient must try to remain peaceful and calm throughout the process of getting treatment.

- The great women in the Bible did not start as great. They each went through something traumatic, heartbreaking, or devastating before they could be perceived as great.

- Friends are wonderful to talk to, and it is therapeutic to have someone to express feelings, but when there is no friend around, you can pray and cry out loud to your constant Friend, God.

# Chapter 5

## Comforting Words for the Soul

*Everyday is a miracle; some days they're just bigger than normal.*

*~ Billy Campbell*

The Holy Spirit of God is Christ personified in the earth realm. After the ascension of Christ into heaven, He left us a Comforter, a guide, a teacher, which is His precious Holy Spirit; and if we are obedient to His leading, we will be blessed because He leads us according to God's will. There will be times when the Holy Spirit will come and specifically give you directions to carry out an assignment. When that happens, you must yield to His leading and tarry not. I vividly remember while in my kitchen preparing to cook one afternoon, I heard a voice inside me say, *I want you to pray for Shod's wife and lay your hands on her stomach. The healing I have given to you, will transfer to her through you to make her uterus strong so she could carry a baby.* The voice was very clear, but I did not know where it was coming from initially. I looked around. No one was there, then I heard the command again. Immediately, I knew it was the voice of God speaking to me.

*Comforting Words for the Soul*

My first thought was *I can't do that. I don't know her that well.* Since I'm not a minister, pastor, evangelist, or any of that, I was wondering why God called me, but I was still going to be obedient, even though I was a little nervous. I had never done anything like that before. I tried to ignore it, thinking that it was my crazy mind and not the Lord, but the voice inside kept telling me to go and pray for her. Shod is my nephew. I attended his wedding, but I really wasn't aquatinted with his wife that well.

    Out of obedience, I called Shod's mother and told her what had happened to me. I told her that I did not think I could do it, and her response to me was, *I can't do this for you. God asked "you" to do it, not me, but I will go with you.* She said that she would call her son Shod and have him give me a call. I told him what the Lord had told me to do. He explained that his wife was at work, but that he would have her to call me. Doris, Shod's mother is a spiritual woman, and I knew that she would give me guidance about my assignment. We called her Sister Barbara, who also was a spirit-filled woman and told her about the assignment. Barbara asked me when was I supposed to return to work. When I told her, she said, *You must do this before you go back to work.* Speaking with Shod's wife, we set up a time for me to come by. As I was leaving the house to go, I

*A Walking Miracle!*

noticed that I had a flat tire. Right then, I knew that my assignment was the will of God because the devil only fights you when there is a victory waiting to be won, but I made it there by riding with someone else. Upon arrival, I explained to Shod's wife, what God had told me to do by laying my hands on her stomach so that she could carry a baby full term. She became extremely emotional. It was at that moment that I found out that she had miscarried two babies. To make matters worse, she worked as a nurse in the maternity ward at a hospital. She was helping to bring babies into the world, but kept losing her own. This had to be emotional turmoil for her. I began praying for her as the Holy Spirit directed me. I placed my hands on her belly and allowed the Lord to speak His words through me in prayer. We rejoiced and celebrated the victory that we knew was already won in the spirit realm. The following year, she gave birth to a beautiful, bouncing baby girl. Prayer creates a new path where the twists and turns turn your stumbling blocks into building blocks. The prayer of faith unlocks doors that would otherwise be closed. We must learn to trust in God's leading through His Holy Spirit at all times and we must carry out the assignment that He gives us quickly.

## Inspiration

    I have come to believe that each of us has a personal calling that is as unique as a fingerprint. We have to discover what God's plan is for us and then share the testimony with others. It is extremely important to let the Holy Spirit lead us in the right direction. When we give all to Him - mind, body, soul, and spirit, we will always be led to victory. There are four words that we must always tell ourselves in times of fear, trouble, and trials, and those four words are: "This too will pass." When it is time to let the bad things go, let them go. Do not hold on to them or allow them to linger. Everything has an expiration date. You simply cannot keep things past their expiration date. Even food items have a date of consumption and if you eat them past their consumption date, you will get sick. It is the same with things, people, and situations. If you allow them to remain when it is time for them to go, you will get sick. Once your trial is over, let it go. If you are too busy holding on to the past, you will not be able to embrace your glorious future. You must surrender your hope and dreams to God and believe that they will come to pass. I have been blessed to be a blessing to others through my testimony, and I am blessed to have come out on the other side. As I look back over my life, I see that God was always there with me. In my

*A Walking Miracle!*

darkness hours, He was there. My spirit was broken when I was diagnosed with cancer, but I am broken no more. That weeping endured only for a night. Now, I look at life differently. I appreciate every moment of every day. The Bible says in Proverbs 16:24 that pleasant words are like sweetness to the soul and health to the bones. Words of encouragement can inspire and have an impact on the lives of others. I use my words to bless and encourage because we all need that. Giving hope and demonstrating my faith in my Maker helps people to keep hope alive.

**Your Uniqueness**

God does everything in each of our lives for a reason. I felt as though I had done something wrong when I was diagnosed, but then I remembered Job. He didn't do anything wrong to suffer the immeasurable loss and affliction that he endured. I know now that I am what God made me. He made me unique and different for His own purpose. You are what God made you as well. You are different from everyone else. This is why we must stop trying to please everyone else and strive to please God. You are different for His purpose, not so that you can fit in with others. There is a reason why you do not fit in. If you are reading this, then that means that you are here on this earth for a reason. God healed me, and if He did it for me, He can do the same for you. You just have to believe and do not doubt. There is no room for doubt. I accept what God had me to go through and I am thankful that He used me. Always inspire and encourage others when you can. Be kinder than necessary because everyone you meet is fighting some kind of battle. Don't give up when it's your time of trial either. Trials keep you strong. Sad moments keep you human. If you give up when its winter, you will miss the promise of your spring, the beauty of your summer and the fulfillment of your fall. Don't let the pain of one season destroy the joy of all the rest. Do not judge the totality of your life by one difficult season. Work through the difficult times, because they come to make you stronger, wiser and to increase your faith. Better times are sure to come. There is a reason for tough times and it's okay to be afraid, but always remember "I AM" is with thee. That's all you need to know. Everyone has a story to tell, but unfortunately not everyone will tell their story. If God has brought you out of your worse test, then why not share it? Why not tell the world what God has done for you? Regardless of what you think, the truth is that your life is not about you and my life is not about me. Our lives are about using what God has given us to impact others. We are not to try to figure out the future. We are to trust in God who holds

*A Walking Miracle!*

the future in His hands. Always thank Him for what He has done, what He is doing, and what He is going to do. He is able to handle all of your problems, your hurts, your desires, your *everything*. He is not only able, but He is also willing to handle it, and waiting for you to give it to him. He is the same yesterday, today, and forever, and if you trust Him, He will not fail you. Sometimes the best things do not happen in an instant, it requires waiting. If you are waiting for God to change something in your life, do not give up. What He has for you is worth the wait. Good things come to those who wait. Don't worry about tomorrow because God is already there and has worked it out. Sometimes you may feel alone, but He says *I will never leave you nor forsake you (Hebrews.13:5b)*. If we are not careful, life can become a pattern of obligations to the job, the spouse, the children, the church, organizations etc. Unfortunately, in the midst of our busy schedules, we can sometimes lose sight of our true calling to live for Christ, but it's never too late to make a difference in our lives or the lives of those around us. Sometimes we just need to stop and be still for a moment in order to listen to the quiet voice from the Lord.

I'm inspired and want to inspire you. My desire is to help motivate and encourage others to walk courageously in their journey and find hope in all things. I believed in my soul that I was going to be healed and would be cancer free. Even though the Oncologist knew how to treat my cancer in the natural by prescribing me the right medications, it was ultimately God, the Great Physician, who healed me. I am God's miracle! As I was walking through my valley of the shadow of death, there were days I would be so down because of all of the appointments or tests, but the scriptures gave me comfort. The following were some of the scriptures that I would read constantly to comfort my soul:

**Proverbs 3:5-6:**
Trust in the Lord with all thine heart; and lean not unto thine own understanding. In all thy ways acknowledge Him, and He shall direct thy paths.

**Romans 8:37-39:**
Nay, in all these things we are more than conquerors through Him that loved us. For I am persuaded, that neither death, nor life, nor angels, nor principalities, nor powers, nor things present, nor things to come, nor height, nor depth, nor any other creature, shall be able to separate us from the love of God, which is in Christ Jesus our Lord.

**Isaiah 55:11:**
So shall my Word be that goeth forth out of my mouth: it shall not return unto me void, but it shall accomplish that which I please, and it shall prosper in the thing whereto I sent it.

**Philippians 4:13:**
I can do all things through Christ which strengthens me.

**Mathew 17:20:**
If ye have faith as a grain of a mustard seed, ye shall say unto this mountain, Remove hence to yonder place; and it shall remove; and nothing shall be impossible unto you.

The scriptures gave me comfort and were like refreshing water to my soul. I was able to make it through another day while reading the scriptures. I would often remind myself of what is written in 2 Chronicles 20:15 which states, *Don't be afraid nor dismayed because of this great multitude, for the battle is not yours, but the Lords.* I kept reminding myself that God is in the midst of it all. God is my Shepherd (Psalms 23). He is in front of us, in back of us, and He is all around us. All day and all night, the angels are watching over us. He wants us to feel the sweetness of His presence.

As a cancer survivor, I still have to go to the cancer center every three months for routine checkups, but now when I go there, I walk tall and proud like a male peacock, colorful, proud, and thankful to know how good God has been to me. This is quite a difference to how I was when I first began going there. I want others to realize that you can live with this disease and live life to the fullest. We must have faith and renewed minds because faith begins within our thoughts.

### Every day is a Miracle

If you believe or have been taught that miracles happen and can occur in your life, then your mind is open to receiving miracles, and they can manifest in your life easily. If you are around people who are constantly speaking, believing, and declaring healing, then you will begin to believe that healing can take place in your life as well. Your faith plays a very important role in the belief system that you hold. You must be positive in order to allow the operation of miracles into your life. When you are positive, you will see that your life will change for the better. Analyze your thoughts on a daily basis. Determine whether the nature of your predominating thoughts is positive or negative. Recognize any hindering thoughts and/or beliefs and replace them with constructive thoughts of faith and courage. When you do this, the influx of miracles will become easier to operate into your life.

### A Visit from the Master Physician

About six months after I had seen the vision of me on a white stallion, I had another experience. This was not a vision, but it was definitely a miracle. I was awakened about 2:00a.m. when I felt a strange sensation in both of my breasts. It felt like a wave of electricity flowing through both of them. Feeling this, I immediately sat up in the bed and began holding them. I knew that I had just been healed! I screamed, *"Thank you Lord! Thank you Lord! Thank you Lord!"* I knew in my soul that from that very moment, I was totally healed. My husband Charles woke up from my screaming and said *"What's wrong?"* I said, *"I've just been healed!"* I knew deep down that God had come to me and healed me. All I had to do was believe, and I did. It was that moment that my faith was taken to another level. I chose to focus on God's promises and the experiences I had just had. I thought that after that night, I would not have to go through anymore treatments, and from that moment, I would need no more doctors, but I came to realize that although I knew I had been healed, my healing took place in the spirit realm first. I had to walk it out by faith in the natural realm. I had to allow time for the spirit to connect to the natural; therefore, I continued going to my doctor's appointments, taking my treatments and doing as I was told, but I knew in my soul that I was only going through the process because I had been healed!

### Miracle on the Hudson

On January 15, 2009, an Airbus A320-214 left LaGuardia Airport headed for Charlotte, North Carolina when they flew into a large flock of Canadian Geese at takeoff. The birds got into both engines and immediately caused engine failure. The pilot had no engine power to make an emergency landing at the nearest runway, and was forced to land in the Hudson River off midtown Manhattan, New York. This incident became known as the "Miracle on the Hudson". The U.S. Airways pilot in command was 57 year-old Captain Chesley B. Sullenberger "Sully", a former fighter pilot who had been an airline pilot since leaving the United States Air Force in 1980. He is also a safety expert and a glider pilot. God, in His divine providence had put

*A Walking Miracle!*

"Sully" on assignment that day. Another pilot may not have been able to make such a landing, but this particular pilot was in the right place at the right time, and had the right skills to make such a landing that resulted in the loss of no lives.

Billy Campbell, a passenger on that plane quoted the following, which resonates within me often: *Every day is a miracle; some days they're just bigger than normal.* Passenger Michele Davis, also a passenger on that plane said, *Every one has a plane crash. You just have to figure out how to deal with it.* Speaking as a walking, talking, living miracle myself, I thank God daily for what He has manifested into my life. Waking up to a brand new day is a miracle, which is a gift from God. That's why we call each day "the present." Life itself is a gift. When you appreciate what you have, and not focus on what you do not have, you will discover that your life is miraculous in so many ways. God works miracles every day. We just do not always recognize them. We must stay motivated and always remember God's grace, mercy, and favor extended to us daily. Being a flight attendant for almost 40 years (as of this writing), I knew when that airplane landed in the Hudson, it was a miracle from God all mighty! Nothing like that had ever happened before. That incident was unprecedented.

*Comforting Words for the Soul*

How wonderful is God? Those passengers were safe not because of the absence of danger but because of the presence of God. His son died in order for us to live, therefore we should be motivated about how much He loves us. Jesus Christ is our example. We cannot avoid being knocked down, but we can decide whether to get knocked out. I was sucker-punched, and afterwards, I fell down, but I was not knocked out. I chose to get up and fight back. I cried out to Him to help me fight and He did. As a result, He healed me. I did not lose my faith, my joy, nor my motivation for life. And what is so miraculous about my story is that I never experienced a day of sickness. I now put all my trust in Him. Do not ever hesitate to ask God for what you need. Ask for spiritual vision to always see Him at work in all things, even what seems to be bad when it comes your way. You must trust Him even when you cannot see Him or feel Him, knowing He causes everything to work together for good to those who love Him and are called according to His purpose (Roman 8:28). When you trust in the Lord and hold on tightly to your faith without it wavering, the Lord will cause you to drink from your saucer because your cup will overflow.

*A Walking Miracle!*

## Motivation to Live

Fighting cancer caused me to have many overcast days and nights. but miraculously I saw the sun shining bright through the clouds. Because of the rough ride, I know I have a friend in Jesus and I thank God for all of my blessings. My cup now runs over and I am drinking from my saucer, and it is good. As I continue to encourage others of God's awesome power, I will let them know that their cup can overflow too and that it is okay to drink from their saucer. Remember when praying, we have a responsibility to seek His will. Our wish is not always His command when it is not aligned to His will for our lives. Praying to God is having an intimate relationship with Him. When we pray and ask for good health, financial needs, relationship harmony etc. remember that we are talking to someone who loves us and who desires the best for us. He knows what we really need before we ever ask. However, He wants us to ask because that is what having relationship with Him is. The quality of any relationship is the quality of the communication. Try to avoid going to God with a wish list and go to Him just because He is God. Have a heart of thanksgiving and gratitude and express that to Him. When you focus solely on His love, everything else you desire will fall into place when it is according to His will. We do not brag about our love for God; we brag about His love for us. He loves us unconditionally and when we turn our heart towards Him just because we love Him, great and mighty things will happen, including healing in all areas of your life. I am motivated to continue on this journey of faith, miracles, and positive thinking.

The diagnosis was difficult for me, however God strengthened my character, my spirit, and my soul giving me motivation to help give my testimony and draw me Closer to Him and His people. I have learned to deal with the good, the bad, and the ugly. When I wake up each morning, I sit on the side of my bed and say, *Thank you Lord, for waking me up today.* I have been constantly reminding myself that I am just a human being. I cannot do everything, but I can get closer to God and love Him more by loving others as He does. Life is unpredictable and fragile. We are given one breath at a time, and one heartbeat at a time, so when death comes to one of us, it affects all of us because the realization that we must all leave this earth is one from which we can't escape. God did not make Pat Johnson a wife, a mother, a grandmother, a friend, a sister, an auntie, etc. just for the sake of having roles; but He made me a woman who is strong, confident, and proud. He made a woman who loves Him, His people, and His Word. We all have roles, but within those roles, we have a responsibility to God in each of those roles. Our roles define us on the outside, but not necessarily on the inside. It is ultimately our devotion to God and His love for us that truly defines who we are.

    In order to stay balanced sometimes, we must be like a ballerina focusing our minds and eyes on one spot to maintain balance. If we focus on circumstances, we will become dizzy and confused. We must lean on God and He will keep our steps steady. He is the focal point in our lives. He will refresh our thoughts and renew our thinking. If at times you feel like a spinning top whirling around and around, then the way to keep your balance is to fix your eyes on God. That is the answer to everything in life. Cancer has shown me how to be motivated for life! I have taken something that was life-threatening, devastating, and scary as hell and turned it into something that I can use to help myself live life to the fullest. Additionally, I can now show other people how to do the same no matter what life has thrown their way. God knows what is in your heart, and He knows what you need before you ask. Even when you do not know for sure, God knows, because He knows you better than you know yourself. He knows the outcome of every situation, and He's guiding you, even when you might feel that you have lost your way. He knows how much you can bear, and

*Comforting Words for the Soul*

He will give you strength, fill you with grace, and give you power and peace as He walks with you every step of the way. He is surrounding you with His love and holding you gently in the palm of His hand. Songwriter and singer Marvin Sapp has a song entitled, 'My Testimony' that I would listen to in order to uplift my spirit. Some of the lyrics in that song are, *I made it through. I am still alive and I am still standing. I have some scars, but I'm still alive. In spite of the storm and rain, heartache and pain, I made it through.* As I listen to that song, I feel that it was written and sang just for me. My hope and dream is to leave this world where there is no more cancer. This experience has led me to help others. I talk to strangers in the mall, grocery stores, and beauty salons letting them know how important it is to get their mammograms every year because early detection is the key to survival. I even stress to men to be checked regularly for prostate cancer, and I pass out literature and information about cancer in general.

### Trusting Against all Odds!

With experiences should come wisdom, and with wisdom should come humility. I thank God for both. Confessing that I have wisdom may not be humble to some, but refusing to accept what you know you have is false

*A Walking Miracle!*

humility. Jesus said, *I am the light of the world. A city that is set upon a hill cannot be hid (Mathew 5:14).* His light dwells within me and I walk in the light as He is in the light. His love and light radiates through me emanating from my soul and I am full of joy indeed! I refuse to hide my light because He has given it to me to dispel darkness and I do that by encouraging others and spreading my testimony. He is the light of today, tomorrow, and yesterday and He is the light in you. There is no other like Him. Embrace the light.

If you are anything like me, you have prayed and asked God to take away your troubles and bad times. I have asked more than once, twice, and three times. But sometimes we need those troubles to teach us faith in Him. Man says, *Show me and I will trust you,* but God says, *Trust me and I will show you.* Our calling is to trust God no matter what it looks like. When things are good, trust Him. When things are bad, trust Him. When things are in-between, trust Him. He is always there, even when you feel you do not have the strength to carry on. Trust me, I have been there. Again I asked, what would you do if you were told you have stage four breast cancer and that the cancer was in your spine, your hip, your breast, your lymph nodes, and your bones. That was me, so I think I am well qualified to tell you that God will never leave you when you totally trust Him. Give everything to Him, and leave them there. I had two choices, I could have given up to cancer or rely on God. I decided to rely on God; therefore, the battle was not mine, but His. As I look back now, I realize how high I have been elevated spiritually as I remember how low I had been mentally.

### Tenaciously Pink

As I stated earlier, it is extremely important to have a support system of family and friends around you to help build you up when you feel that you are falling. My church was extremely supportive of me as I was going through this struggle of fighting breast cancer. They walked with me from the beginning of my journey until the day I announced that I was cancer-free. As a result, I was asked to start a cancer awareness group. I had to think of a name for the group, so I went home and talked to my husband Charles about it. He said to me, *You are a tenacious woman. Look up the word tenacity and see if that fits.* When I looked it up, I discovered that it meant to 1. stick with something 2. to never give up, even when times get tough, and 3. to never surrender; After looking up the definition, I said to him, *How did you come up with this word? It's powerful!* and He said, *Trisha when you were diagnosed, I couldn't believe how you handled it, and I said to myself, This woman has*

*A Walking Miracle!*

*tenacity.* He said, call it 'Tenaciously Pink.' That is how I came up with the name of my Breast Cancer Awareness Group at the church. It brought to mind the popular saying: *When life throws you lemons, make lemonade!* At each meeting, we serve pink lemonade and I love drinking a big, cold glass of lemonade.

## POINTS TO PONDER

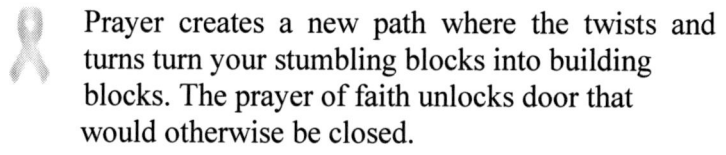

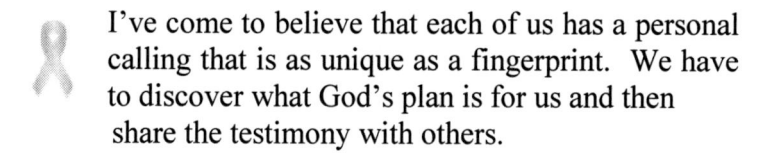

- Prayer creates a new path where the twists and turns turn your stumbling blocks into building blocks. The prayer of faith unlocks door that would otherwise be closed.

- I've come to believe that each of us has a personal calling that is as unique as a fingerprint. We have to discover what God's plan is for us and then share the testimony with others.

- There are four words that we must always tell ourselves in times of fear, trouble, and trials, and those four words are: *"This too shall pass."*

- God's knows what's in your heart and He knows what you need before you ask.

When things are good, trust Him. When things are bad, trust Him. When things are in-between, trust Him. He is always there, even when you feel you do not have the strength to carry on.

# Chapter 6
## Men & Breast Cancer

*When someone has cancer, the whole family and everyone who loves them does, too.*
*~Terri Clark*

I have put this information in the book because it is important that the public understand that breast cancer does not just affect women, but it affects a percentage of men as well, so this information must be shared. Most of what we know about breast cancer is related to women, but it is also prevalent in men. Although breast cancer in men is rare, it does exist. There is still much to learn about breast cancer in men because the percentage in men is so rare, but in the United States, about one percent of all breast cancers occur in men. However, breast cancer rates in men have remained stable over the past 30 years. While there are some similarities between breast cancer in women and men, there are some differences.

**What are the numbers?**
In 2013, it is estimated that among U.S. men there will be:

- 2,240 new cases of breast cancer (compared to 232,340 among women)
- 410 breast cancer deaths in men (compared to 39,620 among women)

**The Male Breast**
Boys and girls begin life with similar breast tissue. Over time, however, men do not have the same complex breast growth and development as women. At puberty, high testosterone and low estrogen levels stop breast development in males. In adult women, breast tissue is a complex network of lobules and ducts in a pattern that looks like bunches of grapes. Lobules are small round sacs that produce milk and ducts are the canals that carry milk from the lobules to the nipple openings during breastfeeding. In men, some milk ducts exist, but they remain undeveloped. Lobules are most often absent.

**Types of Breast Cancer**
For both men and women, most breast cancers begin in the milk ducts of the breast (invasive ductal carcinomas). Fewer than five percent of male breast cancers begin in the lobules. In rare cases, men can be diagnosed with inflammatory breast cancer, or Paget disease of the breast.

*A Walking Miracle!*

**Breast Cancer Screening**

Breast cancer screening tests such as clinical breast exams and mammograms are used to find breast cancer in people with no symptoms. These tests are not recommended for most men. However, some men who have a higher risk of breast cancer may benefit from the screening, including those with:

> A mutation in the *BRCA2* or *BRCA1* gene (or a first-degree relative with a mutation)

> A strong family history of breast cancer, such as mother and/or sister diagnosed at age 40 or younger
If you are a male, and have concerns about your risk of breast cancer, please talk to your health care provider.

**Breast cancer screening recommendations for men at higher risk**

The National Comprehensive Cancer Network (NCCN) recommends that men at higher risk for breast cancer do the following:

> Have a clinical breast exam every six to 12 months, starting at age 25

- Consider having a mammogram at age 40 (depending on the findings from this first mammogram and the amount of breast tissue. Yearly mammograms may be recommended)
- Men at higher risk for breast cancer should also be aware of the warning signs of breast cancer listed below.

**Warning signs**

For men, breast cancer most often presents as a painless lump or thickening in the breast. However, any change in the breast or nipple can be a warning sign of breast cancer including:

- Change in the size or shape of the breast
- Dimpling, puckering, or redness of the skin of the breast
- Itchy, scaly sore or rash on the nipple
- Pulling in of the nipple (inverted nipple) or other parts of the breast
- Nipple discharge

If you notice any of these signs or other changes in your breast, chest area, or nipple, please see your doctor right away. Some men may be embarrassed about a change in their breast or chest area and put off seeing a provider, but this may result in a delay in diagnosis. Survival is highest when breast cancer is found early.

**Risk Factors**
Although some factors have been found to increase the risk of breast cancer in men, most men who are diagnosed have no known risk factors (except for older age).

**Age**
Getting older increases the risk of breast cancer. Older age is the most common risk factor for breast cancer in both men and women. In men, most breast cancer occurs between the ages of 65 and 67 (this is a bit older than it is for women).

***BRCA2 Gene Mutations***
Men and women with an inherited *BRCA2* (breast cancer gene 2) mutation have an increased risk of breast cancer. Men can inherit a *BRCA2* mutation from either parent. A man who has a *BRCA2* mutation can pass the mutation on to his children.

Breast cancer in men is more likely than breast cancer in women to be related to an inherited gene mutation. Up to 40 percent of male breast cancers may be related to *BRCA2* mutations, while only five to ten percent of female breast cancers are considered to be due to a gene mutation. It's usually recommended that men diagnosed with breast cancer have genetic testing for possible *BRCA2* mutations. Even among men who have a *BRCA2* mutation, breast cancer is uncommon. Men who carry a *BRCA2* mutation have about a seven percent chance of developing breast cancer by age 70. In comparison, women who carry a *BRCA2* mutation have a 40 to 60 percent chance of developing breast cancer by age 70. Other genes are under study for a possible link to male breast cancer.

### *Family History*
Whether or not a man carries a *BRCA2* mutation, having a family member with breast cancer increases the chances of developing breast cancer.

### **Radiation Exposure**
Exposure to large amounts of radiation early in life (such as radiation treatment for childhood cancer) may increase breast cancer risk.

## Other Risk Factors
Although information is limited at this time, some conditions related to hormone levels in the body are under study for a possible link to breast cancer in men, including the following:

- Enlargement of the breast tissue; the most common benign breast condition in men)
- Heavy alcohol use
- Chronic liver disease
- Obesity
- Some hormone drugs used to treat prostate cancer

## Treatment
Treatment for breast cancer is the same for men and women. It includes surgery (usually mastectomy for men) plus some combination of radiation therapy, chemotherapy, and/or targeted therapy. Because most breast cancers in men are hormone receptor-positive, treatment usually includes hormone therapy with tamoxifen.

## Survival
Breast cancer survival for men is about the same as for women of the same age and cancer stage at diagnosis.

However, men tend to be diagnosed at a later stage than women. This may be because they are less likely to report symptoms. The most important factors related to breast cancer survival for both men and women are tumor size and whether or not cancer has spread to the lymph nodes. The five-year relative survival rate for men with breast cancer is 84 percent. This means men with breast cancer are, on average, 84 percent as likely as men in the general population to live five years beyond their diagnosis. The 10-year relative survival rate for men with breast cancer is 72 percent. Remember, these rates are only averages that vary and depends on each man's diagnosis and treatment.

**Race/ethnicity Differences in Survival**
Similar to women, there appear to be racial and ethnic differences in breast cancer survival rates among men. African American men are more likely to die from their breast cancer than white men. Although data are limited, African American men tend to be diagnosed with larger, later stage breast cancers than white men. The reasons behind these differences are unclear at this time, but this topic is under study.

*A Walking Miracle!*

**Support**
Because most people think of breast cancer as something that only affects women, men who are diagnosed may feel embarrassed or isolated. For example, a man may likely be the only man with breast cancer at his treatment center. These feelings can be hard for friends and family to understand. Finding sources of social support may help. Counseling and other types of support are also available. A health care provider may be helpful in finding these resources. In-person support groups for men with breast cancer can be hard to find. However, there are support groups for men with any cancer diagnosis. And, there may be online support groups where men with breast cancer can share common experiences. Some organizations may even be able to help men with breast cancer connect with other male survivors for one-on-one telephone or online support.

As mentioned, a man being diagnosed with breast cancer is rare, but I personally know a man who was diagnosed with breast cancer. Terrell Thomas was a flight attendant with me from Atlanta, Ga. We became friends, and he soon began calling me his second mother. As such, he calls me every Valentine's Day and every Mother's Day. When I got the call in April of 2009 that he had been diagnosed with breast cancer a year after my diagnoses, I was shocked. He had ignored the lump in his breast and finally decided to go to the doctor to have it checked out. Needless-to-say, that lump was a malignant mass. Terrell was the first man I knew to have had a double mastectomy. Currently, he is doing well, is faithful in taking his tamoxifen, and is cancer free. This chapter is dedicated to him and all men who have been diagnosed with breast cancer. Please men, listen to your body. It will let you know when something is wrong.

The information in this chapter was taken from the Susan G. Komen website at http://ww5.komen.org/Content.aspx?id=19327356734.

### Prayer for Cancer

I once saw an acronym for the letters A.S.A.P: **A**lways **S**ay **A P**rayer. It is written in the book of 1st Corinthians 13:2, the following: ...and though I have the gift of prophecy, and **understand all mysteries, and all knowledge**...and have not charity (love), I am nothing. I have made a point of highlighting that verse because although cancer is a mystery, there is knowledge of a cure in the mind of God, and God will reveal that cure in His own timing. And who knows, maybe He has already revealed the cure to someone on this earth. However, it is important to note that with the revelation of knowledge and the uncovering of mysteries, there must be love for God's people. Some have the knowledge of many things, but because there is no love for people, that knowledge has not been made known. Therefore, below is a prayer for cancer and the prayer was written in love and is to be prayed in love:

*Holy Spirit, reveal the cure for breast cancer and all cancers. Increase the wisdom, knowledge, and understanding of medical doctors, nurses, researchers technicians, and healthcare personnel who conduct cancer studies and administer treatment to breast cancer patients. Fill those who are undergoing cancer treatments with strength, courage, and patience. Strengthen their immune system and protect their bodies as they undergo chemotherapy, radiation therapy, biological therapy, hormone therapy, and other procedures they may be undergoing. Holy Spirit, I ask in love that you comfort their family members and give them peace. Help them to cast their cares upon You, because You are He who cares for us all. Remind their loved ones to have faith and to believe God for healing and a cure. In your holy, sovereign, and righteous name I pray, Amen*

## POINTS TO PONDER

- Breast cancer does not just affect women, but it affects a percentage of men as well.

- In rare cases, men can be diagnosed with inflammatory breast cancer, ductal carcinoma in situ (a non-invasive breast cancer) or Paget disease of the breast.

- For men, breast cancer most often presents as a painless lump or thickening in the breast. However, any change in the breast or nipple can be a warning sign.

- Older age is the most common risk factor for breast cancer in both men and women. In men, most breast cancer occurs between the ages of 65 and 67.

## Scriptures for Healing

### Isaiah 41:10-14 Scripture
Do not be afraid, for I am with you. Do not be discouraged, for I am your God. I will strengthen you and help you. I will hold you up with my victorious right Hand. See, all your angry enemies lie there confused and humiliated. Anyone who opposes you will die and come to nothing. You will look in vain for those who tried to conquer you. Those who attack you will come to nothing. For I hold you by your right hand - I, the Lord your God. And I say to you, Don't be afraid. I am here to help you. Though you are a lowly worm, O Jacob, do not be afraid, people of Israel, for I will help you. I am the Holy One of Israel.

### Scriptural Prayer
I confess that I will not be afraid because God is with me. I will not be discouraged, for the Lord is my God.

If you are afraid and discouraged, be honest with the Lord and tell Him how you are feeling. Then, choose not to be afraid and to be encouraged. Trust the Holy Spirit to replace your fear and discouragement with God's confidence, peace, and joy. God will strengthen you and help you. God will uphold you with His righteous right Hand. This disease will be confused and humiliated. Every demonic attack will be destroyed and come to nothing. I will look in vain for those who tried to conquer me. The Lord my God holds my right hand and I will not be afraid because He has said that He will help me and I believe Him.

### Isaiah 53:4-5
For sure He took on Himself our troubles and carried our sorrows. Yet we thought of Him as being punished and hurt by God, and made to suffer. But He was hurt for our wrong-doing. He was crushed for our sins. He was punished so we would have peace. He was beaten so we would be healed.

### Scriptural Prayer
Jesus carried my sicknesses and pains and it was thought that God was punishing Him for His own sins. But He was pierced for my rebellion and crushed for my sins. Jesus was beaten so that I could be whole and whipped so that I could be healed. I accept what He has done for me and I accept the healing in my body as a result of His sacrifice.

### Mark 11:22-26
Then Jesus said to the disciples, *Have faith in God. I tell you the truth, you can say to this mountain, 'May you be lifted up and thrown into the sea,' and it will happen.* But you must really believe it will happen and have no doubt in your heart. I tell you, you can pray for anything, and if you believe that you have received it, it will be yours. But when you are praying, first forgive anyone you are holding a grudge against, so that your Father in heaven will forgive your sins, too.

As the Holy Spirit brings people to your mind, begin to forgive them in Your heart. Go through this exercise of forgiving until your heart catches up with your mind. In other words, forgive until you know that you are honestly sincere and trust the Holy Spirit to heal any wounds in your soul. For deeply inflicted wounds, consider talking to a Christian counselor who will guide you through your feelings and emotions. If the Holy Spirit prompts you, call or personally speak to those person(s), and let them know that you have forgiven them and have released the offense. If you need to ask someone to forgive you, swallow your pride and ask for forgiveness. The Holy Spirit will help you every step of the way. Because of the redemptive work of Jesus Christ, you are able to forgive and be forgiven. Remember, God has forgiven us of our sins and our offenses are much greater than those we have experienced from other people. If He is willing to forgive us, we must be willing to forgive people. After praying about forgiving others, then pray for healing.

**Scriptural Prayer**
Now that I have taken care of that matter, I want to say that I have faith in God. Therefore, I command this "mountain" of (name the disease) to leave my body and I cast it into the sea. I believe that the command that I have spoken will bring healing to my body, now. Father, as You instructed, I choose to forgive (name those people) who have offended or hurt me. Holy Spirit, please help me to remember everyone that I need to forgive.

## Healing Affirmations
*With my heart open to God's renewing love,
I accept my healing now.*

*I am healthy and strong because I am one with
God's healing, revitalizing presence.*

*I am created in the image of God, blessed
with strength and wholeness.*

*The power of God sustains and blesses me
with perfect health.*

*I have instant access to God's healing power within.
I am whole and well in mind, body, and spirit.*

### ***Our Deepest Fear***
*"Our deepest fear is not that we are inadequate. Our deepest fear is that we are powerful beyond measure. It is our light, not our darkness that most frightens us. We ask ourselves, Who am I to be brilliant, gorgeous, talented, and fabulous? Actually, who are you not to be? You are a child of God. Your playing small does not serve the world. There is nothing enlightened about shrinking so that other people won't feel insecure around you. We are all meant to shine, as children do.*

*We were born to make manifest the glory of God that is within us. It's not just in some of us; it's in everyone. And as we let our own light shine, we unconsciously give other people permission to do the same. As we are liberated from our own fear, our presence automatically liberates others."*

~Marianne Williamson

## About the Author

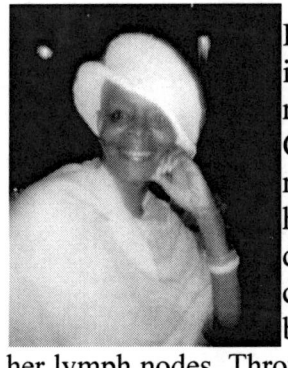

Patricia Johnson was born and raised in Miami, Florida where she matriculated in the Miami-Dade County Public School System. She is married to Charles Johnson, and they have two adult sons. In 2008, Pat was diagnosed with stage four breast cancer. The cancer was in her left breast, her hip, her spine, and her lymph nodes. Throughout her process of treatments, she never had a day of physical pain, no sickness, no chemotherapy, and no radiation, AND she is cancer free today!

Patricia lives her life spreading the news to cancer patients that they can beat it. Cancer does not have to be your death sentence. She also encourages young women to get their annual mammograms. Pat is an inspiration and ray of sunshine to all she encounters. She wrote this book to be a source of encouragement to both men and women with cancer.

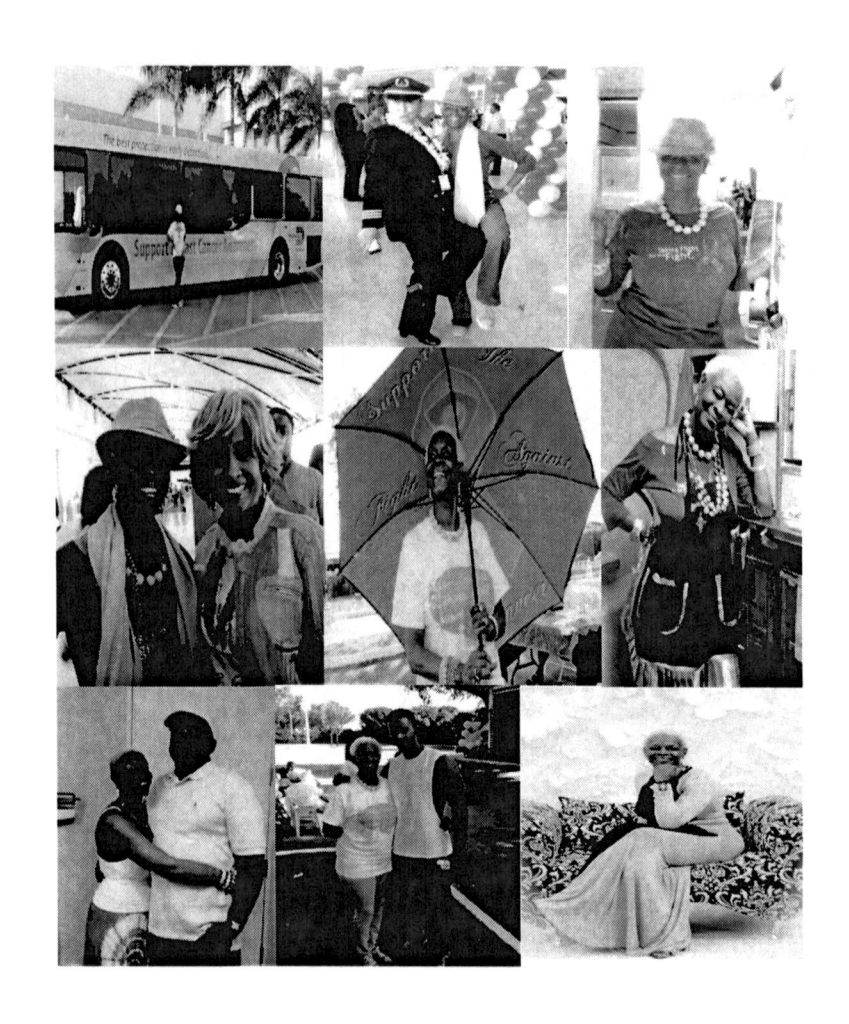

CPSIA information can be obtained at www.ICGtesting.com
Printed in the USA
LVOW12s1913111113

360818LV00001B/3/P